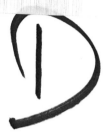

The Secret of Perfect Vision

The **Secret** of
Perfect Vision

How You Can
Prevent or Reverse
Nearsightedness

David De Angelis

Foreword by Dr. Lee Anthony De Luca

Afterword by Otis Brown

Berkeley, California

Published by
North Atlantic Books
P.O. Box 12327   Cover and book design by Jan Camp
Berkeley, California 94712

Printed in the United States of America

The Secret of Perfect Vision: How You Can Prevent and Reverse Nearsightedness is sponsored by the Society for the Study of Native Arts and Sciences, a nonprofit educational corporation whose goals are to develop an educational and crosscultural perspective linking various scientific, social, and artistic fields; to nurture a holistic view of arts, sciences, humanities, and healing; and to publish and distribute literature on the relationship of mind, body, and nature.

MEDICAL DISCLAIMER: The following information is intended for general information purposes only. Individuals should always see their health care provider before administering any suggestions made in this book. Any application of the material set forth in the following pages is at the reader's discretion and is his or her sole responsibility.

North Atlantic Books' publications are available through most bookstores. For further information, call 800-733-3000 or visit our website at www.northatlanticbooks.com.

Library of Congress Cataloging-in-Publication Data

De Angelis, David, 1963–
The secret of perfect vision : how you can prevent and reverse nearsightedness / by David De Angelis.
     p. cm.
     Summary: "Presents a scientifically supported system that directly intervenes with the causes that generate myopia onset and development, and provides exercises that lead to the gradual strengthening of one's focusing capability and the gradual decreasing of refractive error"—Provided by publisher.
     Includes bibliographical references and index.
     ISBN 978-1-55643-677-2
     1. Visual training. 2. Myopia—Alternative treatment. 3. Eye—Refractive errors—Alternative treatment. I. Title.
RE960.D4 2008
617.7'5—dc22

                                                                    2007039566

1 2 3 4 5 6 7 8 9 Sheridan 14 13 12 11 10 09 08

I dedicate *The Secret of Perfect Vision* to those people
who—through their faith and perseverance—will succeed
in improving and ending their refractive errors; to the men and
the women whose personal example and testimony
can free future generations from wearing glasses, contact lenses,
and other ophthalmologic devices, which will
finally be seen as artificial and barbaric remedies.

In addition, I dedicate the book to the ophthalmologists
and optometrists who will consider it part
of their jobs to discuss preventive work
and the natural cure of refractive errors.

Contents

Foreword

I've had the great pleasure to meet David De Angelis by accident after having read his book. An ophthalmologist myself, I already knew a lot about the issues his book deals with, but it was amazing to learn about the author's personal experience. His "ex-myope's experience" was incredibly interesting to me.

Despite the fact that David isn't a physician, during our meetings I could see how vast his knowledge about sight is, thanks to his having read and studied specific medical literature. His experience is a clear and perfect example of being able to reach unexpected targets, putting into practice the synthesis of his bibliographic research. He wasn't ready to surrender and accept only what the scientific-medical establishment states on the issue.

Worldwide, famous scholars have been doing research on refractive errors and especially on myopia for years. Unfortunately, a great deal of medical literature has always paid more attention to correcting visual defects rather than looking for their causes and intervening against them. Much work in ophthalmology development today has been dictated by economic interests, so that the greatest scholars have withdrawn from research on alternative methods that could control and even prevent the onset and development of myopia. The studies on visual treatments have been carried out since the early twentieth century, when ophthalmology became a real science. Unfortunately, after so many years, still only traditional correcting methods are offered for myopathy. Ophthalmologists have little interest in proposing alternative methods because it's much easier to prescribe a pair of glasses and it's more profitable to suggest refractive surgery treatment. On the other side, many opticians are interested only in selling ocular prostheses. In some cases the optometrists themselves, the professionals who cure functional disorders that hinder correct eye functioning, don't care about this delicate issue. Our unique hope is that very soon, all the efforts of those who are interested in healing sight may converge to give people a chance of pursuing different, more "natural" but efficacious ways to control or prevent myopia development—the ways that are neglected at present because of personal advantage, profit, or whatever else.

I'm sure that (also thanks to David) visual therapy will continue to develop and will meet the needs of people who have realized how harmful modern society is for eye health. Together with David and all the others who are willing to take a part in this great challenge, I will work hard on spreading and acknowledging the principles and theories that are basic for clear, distinct vision.

—Dr. Lee Anthony De Luca, ophthalmologist

Preface

I am neither an ophthalmologist nor an optometrist.

My friend, the book you are holding in your hands is the fruit of my passion for understanding the visual mechanisms of the eye. This understanding includes the dynamics of healing visual errors. It is the fruit of my personal experience and theoretical knowledge. I have had a great formal education, but some ideas and concepts must develop outside "the ivory towers." In this sense, you learn by doing—which is how I did it. A great deal of direct experimental data suggests the nature of the expected solution, but you must incorporate this knowledge in *your* work to clear your distance vision.

If you are looking for detailed and direct academic certifications to justify your work in using the methods explained in this text, I recommend viewing the following websites:

> www.powervisionsystem.com
> (official website)

> www.powervisionforum.com
> (Power Vision System Support Forum)

> www.chinamyopia.org
> www.myopia.org
> www.myopia-manual.de
> www.myopiafree.com

If you are ready to listen to the voice of someone who once suffered from the frustration of not seeing distant objects clearly, then please take the time to assess the contents of this book.

My Story

I knew I could do it, sooner or later.

I knew that nothing is impossible for the one who *believes* he can do it.

I knew that one day I would get my clear sight back and I would succeed in seeing with my own eyes. I had faith that I could do this without becoming a slave to minus-lens glasses. I knew that I would see all the fantastic details and colors (that a nearsighted person can only imagine) without the "chains" of minus-lens glasses.

Up to the age of fifteen I was normal (so-called emmetropic). I had perfect sight or the proverbial 6/6 or 20/20 vision. For some reason, I began to become myopic, and I was prescribed my first pair of minus-lens glasses. Like many nearsighted people, I got into an intellectual "tunnel in the fog."

This is the situation in which you get caught up in using increasingly stronger and stronger minus-lens glasses—inevitably and inexorably leading to an ever-increasing degree of nearsightedness. I could never stand the glasses. I have always had a physiological rejection of them and judged them as something that did not belong on my face. Above all else, I was certain that I could restore my vision—somehow—despite the fact that I did not know how to do it at the time.

During those years I evaluated everything, groping in the fog of my myopia for a better solution. The fact that I was myopic, compounded by the distorted opinions I was given by eye health professionals, was frustrating and suffocating me.

I read over and over again thousands of books on the issue of "improving your sight." I attempted to use the proposed techniques many times. I tried to understand the mechanisms of correct vision, asking people who could see well what was going on at the moment when they were focusing on something. I was obsessed and fascinated at the same time.

I tried various methods of visual reeducation, including the expensive Accommotrac Vision Trainer (explained more fully later). Though I had gone down this path a thousand times, the results were practically nothing. I was losing my trust in the possibility that somewhere and somehow I would find the correct solution. However, I did not give up hope. I started trusting in science again and continued with my studying.

I have left behind the "fog" of –2.25 and –2.00 diopters (D) of myopia.

A friend of mine once said, "The time comes for the one who knows how to wait." The time comes for the one who knows to wait, how to persevere, and has faith. To this I add, "Sooner or later the solution comes." This solution will look like an unexpected prize. Actually, the solution is open to you if you believe in scientific truth and in the ability to solve problems. I prepared this book as a technical guide and a testament. I also wrote it for open-minded people who wish to follow my path out of myopia.

I know perfectly well that I am going against the present therapeutic theory (Donders-Helmholtz) concerning visual errors. These errors include myopia and farsightedness. I feel my mission is to spread the knowledge that will make people cry in joy at their restored vision—even if it means going against the present establishment in optometry and ophthalmology. I do not enjoy doing this, but sometimes fundamental change requires that we learn how to stand and fight.

Those of you who proceed with trust and perseverance will see with your own eyes flashes of clear vision, and in this process will recognize a gradual improvement in your vision. It is my responsibility to promulgate the scientific truth that will make you free of minus-lens glasses for nearsightedness.

I spent about twelve years of my life looking for and experimenting with various methods to heal my nearsightedness. I had always believed that I would be able to eventually clear my distance vision. I traveled in the fog of doubts that traditional optometry instilled in me. This is the "science" that insists that nothing could be done and that prevention would always be impossible. I was expected to accept this point of view as though there were objective facts to back up this opinion. I learned later that quite a few optometrists themselves believe that prevention is possible by the proper understanding and aggressive use of the plus lens—for prevention.

I have always believed in the possibility of healing our bodies and empowering ourselves as individuals to take control and solve the problem of nearsightedness. It takes a transformation in you if this goal is to be achieved. In order to "cure" someone's physical sight, it is necessary to change his or her internal visualization and understanding of the necessity of prevention. We are all searching for means to heal ourselves at many levels, whether we are aware of it or not.

What I Learned from My "Ex-Myopia"

Myopia has been a great lesson in life for me and is a source of an important education. Restoring my natural sharp sight— by studying—has led me to profoundly change my attitude in many different ways. Even my interaction with people has greatly improved.

The process of renewing my sight has led me to see and understand a great many academic and scientific issues that I was not interested in earlier. Most important, it has helped me cure and heal my relations with many other people. I understood that I was the one who had created, by myself, a barrier that blurred my sight, separating me from others.

This personal insight may sound strange in a book that presents a scientific approach to the cause of myopia. The work that I did on myself, on my eyes and my growing awareness, has led me to an improved sense of perception—of myself and the entire world. If you take this method seriously, heading through the fog of your own vision and doubts, you too will become able to receive the benefits, which could be useful in all your lifetime engagements. In the end, life can be seen as a challenge and a great adventure. It leads you to see your secret desires becoming reality—not only to develop clear distinct sight, but to also become stronger in order to face your doubts and uncertainties.

I'm overjoyed because of the collateral effects of this body of work that I call "The Power Vision System." I chose this name because of its reference to inner vision improvement and to the awareness of our personal wishes—deeply hidden desires that need to evolve and help us realize our potential (beyond improving and strengthening our sight from strictly the physical point of view).

I have defeated my myopia, which has always been considered "incurable" by traditional Western medicine. This has caused me to think over the real possibilities in healing someone—beyond the limits of what was previously thought to be possible that have been set by present traditional medicine. I'm sure that medical science, if it were more interested in the patient's feelings and emotions, could see him or her as a multilevel unity (physical, mental, emotional, spiritual) and could lead us to better results that would surpass merely eliminating or suppressing the symptom. From this viewpoint, a message from our body and soul can move us toward real healing.

What might be the possibilities for a person who restores his own health and, above all, achieves a complete recovery (meant as a total and deep state of well-being and psychophysical harmony)? One's horizon moves toward the harmony of one's being, beyond anyone's expectations. Above all else, ordinary people like you and me, who are always focused on their own little worlds, might be able to solve their major problems. Therefore, I thank my ex-myopia for having given me a chance to embrace myself and my deep desires, as well as for having encouraged me to understand the beauty and the pleasure of giving to myself the images that are reflected in my own eyes.

Bucking Conventional Wisdom

The intellectual resistance most of us put up to innovative ideas is partly caused by the fact that these ideas challenge previous statements that were regarded as "proven." These beliefs have been approved (by some "experts") as unchangeable and eternal. These doubtful statements ("the eye does not change") have become dogma that nobody dares to question.

The new facts are often not easily accepted since they challenge our preconceived notions, which are at the base of the simplistic idea that the eye cannot change. Science is an evolutionary process, and new facts must be recognized and accepted. If we deny this process, then we only perpetuate old problems with intellectually binding dogma of the past. Confining a science within accepted theories means limiting the evolution of fundamental science and research.

The suffocating effects of accepting conventional wisdom without asking questions are well known. Albert Einstein once said something along the lines of, "Imagination is more powerful than knowledge." This statement is warning us not to close our minds to our objections to the traditional (minus-lens) method of optometry. We must expand our knowledge of the dynamic behavior of the eye. This expansion must be on the basis of deeper insight, which necessarily must challenge the current dogma of "standard practice."

The present method of dealing with refractive errors ("make it sharp instantly") seems to be closed and, in my opinion, obsolete. The intellectual resistance to these new ideas comes partly from idleness. But it also comes from the fact that this new concept could disturb already established intellectual authorities and their material positions.

In my judgment, the idea of treating refractive errors under the present (Donders-Helmholtz) system by using corrective lenses is completely out of date. The method and theory are inadequate in light of the large body of existing scientific data that demonstrates that the eye's refraction power "follows" its visual environment. The classical theory insists that the eye is not capable of doing this. The experimental data says that this is exactly the case with the natural eye when it is explicitly tested.

The duty of medicine is to be at the service of people's health. This being the case, the medical community must take into account these facts and seek to understand newer methods. In that manner we can work together toward a better solution and cure.

Obfuscation and authoritarianism are not the proper role of science. These words and attitudes are still alive—and will not help us in the process of developing true knowledge of the eyes' behavior by rational analytic means. Each one of us must be aware of our distance vision and take on the responsibility to maintain clear distance vision and health. Each one of us must be prepared to intervene when required. As for this issue, each one of us could do a great deal on the preventive level. Thus we must learn to share responsibility with others who wish to help us with the preventive process. This must be done before significant negative refractive errors have developed. By this process, you can protect yourself from overaccommodative stress—produced by a confined environment compounded by a strong negative lens—simply by using positive lenses at near distances.

I hope my book can help you open your eyes to the real possibilities of prevention. I believe that in many cases you can cure yourself of functional refractive errors—that is, you can clear your distance vision to normal by using my method.

All nearsightedness is still defined as "incurable" unless you use the palliative of a negative lens. I believe that a great change is developing in this field—where the objective is to free your eyes from nearsightedness. This belief comes through a complete evaluation of the experimental data that demonstrates the true behavior of your eyes. You should widen your own views in the light of the results of these newer scientific truths. I am willing to help you.

My friend, if you have a glint of faith in your mind, and if you follow the instructions in this book, you might well find a new way of seeing. It is possible that a new world is waiting for you at this moment. Trust in your own path of recovery and transformation.

To You, My Dear Friend, Who Has Decided to Change

My dear friend and reader, I know very well each single step you'll make toward improving your vision and getting back your clear sight. I know each level of frustration you'll feel in different moments along your way. I know how much strength you'll need to trust in being able to continue and how much perseverance you'll have to maintain throughout the time.

Each of us tends to stay in our own conditions: emotional, financial, professional. It's hard to be courageous enough to change ourselves. Well, my dear friend, what I can grant you is this: If you are able to be constant in doing the proposed exercises and overcome the "fogging" that follows each flash of clear vision, you will make it work out. You'll reach a level of improvement that lets you understand that it's only a matter of time before you restore your sight completely.

I believe that the real magic of life is in doing something at an artistic level. A system of teaching exists for each kind of art, even for the ability to see clearly. When we were younger, Nature taught us about this ability; unfortunately, many of us have lost it, often because of misusing this extraordinary medium—our eyes.

This is the essence of many psychosomatic diseases and functional disorders: it's not the organ that is ill, but the way we use it. Ancient medicine stated that "the function makes the organ," and the Power Vision System is based on such a statement; reeducating the eyes and giving our best doesn't mean victory at the Olympic Games but getting or getting back the ability to see the world in all its bright and clear beauty.

In this time of open information, we have the capability to overcome limits of distance and meet the masters of specific disciplines. Thanks to the Internet, we have access to those who have studied and experimented for years and years, trying to improve their own sight remarkably. There's a suitable method for everything; it's only a matter of finding a person who's ready to teach you. We must find the key principle for what we are looking for and use it correctly.

You work this system in the following way: to embrace passionately what you really want, really believe in, and keep going with it, until one day, the obstacle (the problem itself) falls down in front of your eyes. Once, somebody wrote, "You must believe in something so as to see it," and I can't think of a better formula for being successful in working with the Power Vision System as well as in life itself.

I'm sure that when you get your clear, distinct vision back, your motivation will grow enormously and you will look for other challenges in your life. Each of us must give something, and we must use our lives as a precious source so as to improve and, whenever possible, give something of ourselves to life and posterity. I dream of that future when many people will be able to make themselves free and be able to take the advantage of this and other similar books that were written with the aim of sight improvement and sustained clear vision for life.

When someone understands the power of changing herself, she is reborn again in a new life, full of hope, motivation, and dreams that one day she could be the master of her body, thanks to faith and trust. We weren't born to suffer, but to learn, grow, and enjoy this life.

Magic, beauty, richness, love, friendship, clear and distinct sight, and whatever else gives you zest for life is at your disposal. The price to pay is the price of commitment: to sail over the troubled waters of doubts, when results come late; to go ahead through darkness; to decide to get out of that flat life.

My dear friend, nothing is impossible if you believe you can make it work.

To the Skeptics in the Scientific Community

A system for treating the undesired refractive states of the eye is not likely to be readily accepted by a great many people in the scientific and/or medical community—but that is not important to the people who have started to see more clearly with their own eyes and without wearing minus glasses or contact lenses. The validity of any preventive or curative technique is based on direct proof with patients and on a strong scientific basis.

There are scientists who believe in this preventive method by use of a plus lens, and have used it successfully on their own eyes to clear their distance to normal. Further, there are people in the medical community who recommend preventive methods as a second opinion.

To all those who have doubts about the Power Vision System (PVS) and its validity in the gradual clearing of myopia and other visual disorders, I ask that they provide the following rationale:

1. Prove that overaccommodative stress, which is driven by excessive accommodation at nearwork, doesn't increase accommodative strength, bringing about a worsening (negative change) in sight.

2. Prove that wearing minus glasses and contact lenses doesn't bring about accommodative increase in muscle tone, therefore worsening sight.

3. Prove that the SAID (Specific Adaptation to the Imposed Demand) Principle does not work well for structural and

functional adaptation of the visual organs. Prove that muscular training and training with blur-driven accommodation, wearing "preventive" lenses (which the Power Vision System is based on) doesn't create adaptation of the eye's refractive status on the basis of the SAID Principle.

4. Explain the reasons why a myopic person is obliged to wear stronger and stronger minus lenses. This is different from the fact that the very same person has become used to wearing the current minus lenses and therefore the current overaccommodative state necessarily worsens his sight.

I hope that I will be able to find scholars within the scientific communities of engineering, ophthalmology, and optometry to back up the Power Vision System and my theories in order to wake up those employed in those sectors and to help the people who have the motivation to reduce or end their dependency on minus-lens glasses or contact lenses. Our goal is to help them clear their sight—gradually and naturally.

My advocacy will likely change the optical business from its traditional practice of using a minus lens. I believe that every physician ought to help his patient in understanding alternative methods—specifically helping him to recover from this "disease"—and not inadvertently make the patient part of an "assembly line" by using a minus lens on great numbers of children and adults. Many patients are not even aware of the potential for effective prevention, because no one has provided them with this critical information. If a patient is on the threshold of nearsightedness, our method could be very effective in a relatively short period of time.

I hope you are willing to join us in this important mission and will help us spread the word about the principles and concepts of healing to the people who have the greatest need for them. I am at your disposal to test and prove the validity of PVS in practice—offering its use in a monitored and controlled study. Our intention is to have the application of this concept applied by serious and motivated scholars, engineers, pilots, and scientists in the field—those who have the greatest need for it.

Introduction

The Power Vision System (PVS) is not a method but a preventive system for you if you are looking for a *valid, effective,* and above all else, *permanent* alternative to wearing glasses.

Myopia often begins as a bad habit. This reality is understood by bioengineers and other scientists. Some optometrists and ophthalmologists have begun to advocate "prevention," but they understand the practical difficulties of putting the preventive method into effect.

The process of seeing is a complex interactive system. This system requires precise coordination of the ocular muscles (those around the eyeball) and specifically of the ciliary muscle. The traditional point of view is fixed on the concept that the ciliary muscle is the only one responsible for the process of accommodation. In my opinion, other factors are involved. The eye is affected by many things, including the extrinsic ocular muscles of the eye as well as by the emotions. The emotions must be considered as an element responsible for one's health, as part of modern psychology and medicine.

We should understand that it is possible to strengthen one's own focusing capability. This includes the possibility of regaining the sight that was lost in years of thoughtless use of our eyes in near-viewing and the compounding effect of strong minus-lens glasses.

The physiological principles are clear. The first among them is the SAID (Specific Adaptation to the Imposed Demand) Principle, fully illustrated as it concerns the use of the visual organs.

A fascinating characteristic of initial success is that preliminary success can be *multiplied,* provided you are willing to learn "winning rules of the game." By reading about and, above all else, *using* the "winning rules" of the Power Vision System, you can gradually decrease the dioptric power of your lenses. The Power Vision System will also help the most confident and persevering of people to reach complete remission of their refractive error.

You will discover a surprisingly clear and vivid world again. Additionally, you will learn a great lesson in life: that everything can come to he who believes he is able to accomplish the task. This awareness will give you power in other fields of endeavor, and you will become free from the unreasonable constraints that each of us creates in our own minds.

Why I Wrote This Book

The Power Vision System is a concentrate of my study and search to resolve my own myopia. The techniques and the illustrated principles can be also used for curing other visual errors. This book represents joy and satisfaction for all those people who really want to *see*. It is the fruit of my own developing knowledge and experience. This knowledge came from reading many books and scientific studies. Further, this knowledge was put into practice by trial and error—based on endless hours of hard work. I went through long periods of deep discouragement and frustration in trying to understand where, why, and how I was making specific mistakes.

After all this work, I now lay my experience at your feet. I have restored my vision, but this goal is not enough for me. My deeper goal is to transfer this knowledge to you. This is the real reason I wrote this book—to help heal your sight.

My friend, I like to think that one day, when you see a flash of clear vision and as your sight starts improving, you will think of me. Perhaps I will also become a part of every view, every landscape you will enjoy seeing with great clarity. I would feel guilty if I kept this knowledge to myself. So, consider this book as my gift and contribution to you.

What This Book Can Do for You

Using the Power Vision System, you can achieve the following results:

- A remarkable increase of visual acuity and a decrease in functional visual errors—including their total elimination—as personally demonstrated by the author.

- A decrease of the diopter power of your present prescription (whether contact lenses or minus-lens glasses). You will become less dependent on them, including the possibility of passing a required eye test—thus eliminating the need for any use of the minus lens.

- An increase in the strength and flexibility of your ocular musculature.

- Better coordination of your eyes. This work will produce a remarkable decrease of strabismus—up to its complete remission and disappearance.

- Better vision for your eyes by reducing visual stress.

Keep in mind: The effort and the time needed to achieve any improvement depends on correct and constant use of the method.

It means that two people with the same visual error can develop noticeably different improvements. This depends on the *quantity* and *quality* of the job they are doing. This specific work is completely described in considerable detail.

The Power Vision System is dedicated to people who are highly motivated to get better sight—up to the gradual disappearance of their visual error. *No one* can replace your own judgment and persistence.

How to Use This Book

The Power Vision System aims at preventing *and reversing* refractive errors. It is primarily addressed to the person who suffers from functional refractive errors like myopia and farsightedness, since the principles of the cures are the same.

I made every effort to analyze all the factors that affect accommodation. They include myopic and hyperopic defocus and the physiological effects of the environment on the eye's focal status. I have studied the techniques of changing refractive conditions with lenses as well as the work of oculomotor musculature. These include techniques of healing taken from the principle of homeostasis. Using these concepts, it is possible to control functional refractive errors. I have done my best to explain all the physiological mechanisms of actions and reactions as I understand them.

This is a manual with two levels of information:

1. A simple one, for readers interested in learning the techniques, and

2. A more complex one, to explain for the sophisticated reader the physiology of mechanisms that are the basis of the proposed preventive techniques

The first level is a practical approach that can be used by the average reader without understanding the underlying theory and physiological explanations. The second level is the PVS theory, intended for specialists or people who wish to go into physiological issues in depth.

Also included in the book are a question-and-answer section, appendices with specialized information, a glossary of terms, a complete reference section listing the scientific studies on which various topics explained in the book are based, and other helpful resources.

I hope that specialized readers, and the scholars in the field, will value and use all the information in the text. This book represents my effort to synthesize the disparate pieces of knowledge contained in scientific publications and research into a systematic method of preventing vision loss. This book isn't meant to accuse or criticize traditional optometry but is intended to induce change in the historical methods of eye care. For that reason, I stake a personal testimony on the real possibility of cure and recovery.

No great radical idea can survive, unless it is embodied in people whose lives are the very message itself.
—Erich Fromm

Those who dream by night in the dusty recesses of their mind wake in the day to find that it was vanity; but the dreamers of the day are dangerous men, for they may act their dream with open eyes, to make it possible.
—T. E. Lawrence

A new scientific truth does not triumph by convincing its opponents and making them see the light, but rather because its opponents eventually die, and a new generation grows up that is familiar with it.
—Max Planck

Those who are rigidly committed to one explanation may have their minds opened up by being encouraged to examine things from an alternate perspective.
—Michael J. A. Howe

Chapter 1

The Physiological Bases of the Power Vision System

Accommodative and Focusing Stimuli: The Way Power Vision Acts

The ocular training used in the Power Vision System (PVS) affects stimuli that control accommodation effects due to blurring or incremental retinal defocus. It works by controlling accommodation through the wise use of positive lenses for nearsighted vision and negative ones for farsighted vision. This leads to a process of gradual adaptation by use of these two training stimuli.

Visual (Sagittal) Axis's Convergence

When observing a near object, the visual axis of the eyes must change. This is called "convergence of the visual axis" of the eyes (since they can't stay parallel). This action allows the image on the two retinas to fuse—allowing three-dimensional viewing. This is a continuous process as we look from far to near and vice versa. The detection of the image is by the *central fovea;* this is the retinal part called the "yellow spot" or *macula,* where the image is maintained to achieve sharp focus (see Figure 1.1).

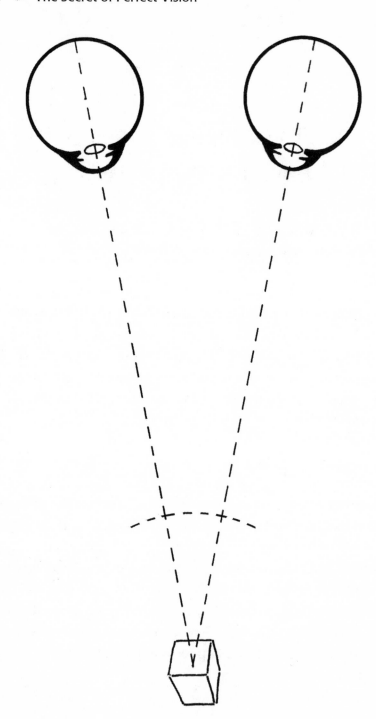

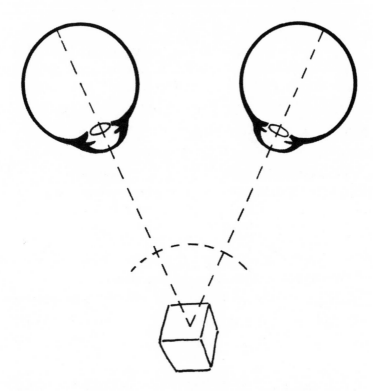

*Figure 1.1   Ocular convergence varies depending on distance
of the observed object.*

Training extrinsic ocular muscles by working at the widest ranges
of their movements, together with the exercises of peripheral fixation (fixing on a point and trying to maintain binocular vision),
is aimed at improving the level of muscular convergence (which
is often jeopardized with nearsightedness at different levels of
strabismus, as the author himself had).

Keep in mind: Peripheral fixation training isn't improving
peripheral vision but the central binocular fixation of an object
or a point that is at extreme parts of the visual field: it has nothing to do with concept of peripheral vision, which means perceiving the objects at the edge of the visual field.

Accommodation: The Way the Eye Focuses

When looking in the distance, the healthy eye (also called *emme-tropic*) focuses light on the retina. In order to focus clearly at near distances, the eye must undergo the process of *accommodation,* where the lens of the eye must change its power proportional to the near distance. This process of accommodation is achieved by the capability of the crystalline lens to change its refractive power to eliminate blur at the surface of the retina. This capability of the eye to vary its focus is completely automatic and involuntary. However, the Power Vision System training allows you to acquire the ability to voluntarily control this process.

The shape of the crystalline lens is changed in order to maintain sharp focus on the retina. This control is exerted by adjusting the ciliary muscle. This is an involuntary muscle; it is under the control of the retina.

Accommodation is controlled by the visual environment. The process of change in the eye is achieved by four interrelated processes. They are:

1. *Accommodation:* A change of power of the crystalline lens; the retina must control this lens to maintain a sharp image on the retina.

2. *Convergence:* Convergence of visual axis is essential. If it does not work properly, you will not achieve a "fused" image. If this system does not work properly, you must use the active ocular stretching exercises that are prescribed in the Power Vision System. Such exercises bring about improvement in both visual function and the focusing system.

3. *Myosis:* This process produces contracting pupils. This is required to modify the depth of field—to achieve sharper focus.

4. *Contracting and relaxing of extrinsic ocular muscles:* By controlling the condition of muscular tonus (contracting and relaxing), the ocular muscles can modify the very sphericity of the eye and therefore "decide" on the point where the focused image will fall. (This statement is not in agreement with the orthodox view on the subject.)

Keep in mind: Functional visual errors depend on conditions of muscular hypercontraction. The muscles in such conditions keep the eye "deformed" perpetually. Therefore this "contraction" does not allow flexible and dynamic use of the structural modifications that are possible. At this point Power Vision System training can help with exercises for the extrinsic ocular muscles.

Central Fovea Focusing

The image must fall at the central fovea. This must happen in order to perceive a perfectly focused image of an object.

The fovea is characterized with a remarkably higher capacity of "performing" the picture. Most of our sharp vision falls within one degree of this structure. Any deviation of the visual axis (even very light strabismus) or, if existing, errors in ocular coordination (binocular visual errors) lead to poor focusing. This is because any imbalance of the extrinsic ocular muscles (just one or both eyes) leads to wrong positioning at the central fovea—therefore causing *retinal eccentricity,* in which retinal receptors (rods and cones) that lie beyond the fovea have a lower capacity of sharp vision (see Figure 1.2). The Power Vision System training overcomes such imbalance by restoring perfect coordination and convergence.

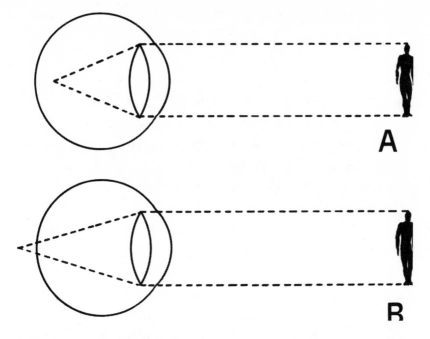

Figure 1.2   The central fovea.

An image must fall at the central fovea, or the most sensitive retinal part, in order for you to perceive a clear image. Any change leads to nonperfect focusing.

A   In the myopic eye, the picture falls in front of the retina. Therefore the image will not be in focus.

B   In the hyperopic eye, the image falls beyond the retina and is out of focus.

Ocular Movements—Rapid Eye Movements

The eye must constantly carry out very rapid movements so as to keep up the continuity of visual perception. Such rapid eye movements are called *saccadic* movements. All the parts of the visual field, when focusing, become made up into one single picture. This capability depends on the level of *ocular dynamic capacity.*

This depends on the extrinsic ocular muscles functioning correctly—and this is a function of their flexibility and strength. A person with functional visual errors has very little ocular mobility, and this is characterized with a "fixed" glance. The Power Vision System restores ocular mobility and dynamics (basics for correct focusing) naturally and gradually.

Binocular and Monocular Vision

Binocular vision acuity is slightly superior to monocular (5–10%). This fact is very important for valuing overaccommodative stress, which is one of the main reasons for the development of myopia.

During a visit to an optometrist, you are often given corrective lenses that are necessary to see the letters at 11/10 ototype with monocular vision. (Instead of 10/11 with binocular vision—that is considered "normal vision." Such lenses would surely cause less overaccommodative stress.) This phenomenon could be easily proven by wearing these prescribed lenses and looking at near objects.

The near objects could be your hands or the floor—both images would be slightly deformed. Ask any optician for an explanation, and you would be told that it is a normal phenomenon and that your eyes must "get used to" the new lenses. Your eyes must adapt (the SAID Principle), generating a very slight myopia to lessen the new lenses' hypercorrection, thus developing a real myopia due to the applied minus lens!

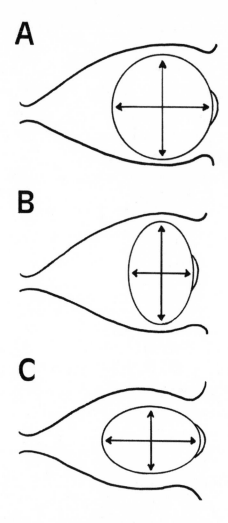

Figure 1.3   Different ocular shapes of the refractive errors.

A. Normal eye: spherical shape—globe.

B   Hyperopic eye: flexibility and strength. The imbalance of the extrinsic muscles deforms the globe of the eye, thus causing inaccurate focus.

C   Myopic eye: hypercontracted extrinsic muscles deform the globe of the eye, causing inaccurate focus.

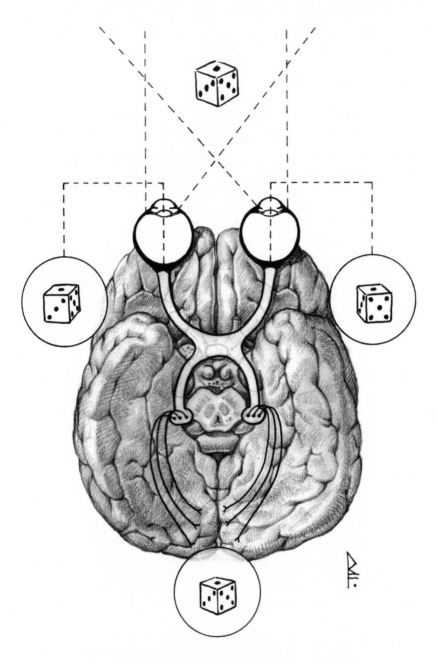

*Figure 1.4   The fusion of the ocular images between
the right and left eye.*

The Etiology (Cause) of Myopia: How You Become Nearsighted

It is necessary to understand the ways you develop myopia, going back to its *causes*. By doing this you will be able to intervene, either in a preventive phase (when myopia is still a temporary defect, so called pseudo-myopia) or in case of fixed myopia, to reduce it.

The development of myopia is attributed to four principal mechanisms:

1. The eye's fundamental proven ability to control its focal status to the visual environment
2. The variations of pressure inside the eye
3. Retinal stretching
4. Retinal defocus

This book deals only with the fourth mechanism (retinal defocus), upon which the Power Vision System is based; the system is exact because of its foundation in this physiological mechanism. This concept is supported by many scientific studies and rehabilitative treatments. (Please see the section "Retinal Defocus and Refractive Change" in Chapter 2 for more details.)

Periods of strong stress produce overaccommodation. This is due to ocular work at excessively near distances. When this happens together with the stress of the *symphatic system,* the result produces an "accommodative spasm." This is described in the scientific literature.

In such cases, accommodation—required when focusing at near distances—becomes greater than normal. For example, to clarify the issue, some children read at variously 4 inches (–10 diopters [D]) and some at 3 inches (–13 diopters). Greater detail in discussing accommodative stimulus is discussed by Suchoff and Petito (1986). Such spasm of accommodation—due to accommodative stress—is seen as kind of adaptation that can cause short periods of retinal defocus.

A person experiences this phenomenon as a fogging of the distance vision. Actually, after shifting her glance from distant to near objects, a person has very weak focus for distant objects. This condition of distant objects' blurring (due to retinal defocus and because of the accommodative spasm) has been researched and classified as nearly 0.2 D (Ehrlinch, 1987; Rosenfield, Ciuffreda, & Novogradsky, 1992) up to 1.00 D (Ong and & Ciuffreda, 1995, 1997). So an increased level of accommodation (say, for example, –13 diopters) creates all the necessary bases for a condition defined as pseudo-myopia to develop.

This "nearsightedness," produced by excessive accommodation, in turn causes instantaneous blurring or myopia. Pseudo-myopia is a condition caused by overaccommodation—actually, a lack of ability to completely relax accommodation. Pseudo-myopia is usually a transitory phenomenon but can in time become permanent if nothing is done to prevent the near environment (Curtin, 1985).

As Young (1971) proposed, the process of developing myopia proceeds in two phases:

1. The first is characterized by a change of accommodative tonus (accommodative spasm due to hyperaccommodation) that makes the ciliary muscle contract.

2. In the second phase, this condition of continuous stress leads to an increase in the globe's axis. This is described as the standard condition of a nearsighted eye.

However, a steady retinal defocus (hyperopic: focus behind the retina) seems to be a precursor for the globe axis's lengthening and therefore is the main reason myopia develops.

Many authors, such as Suchoff and Petito (1986) and Curtin (1985), back up this theory that assumes that retinal defocus is the main stimulus for axial lengthening—and therefore for developing myopia. This theory is based on the assumption that the retina varies its position so as to optimize focusing. This means that the shape of the ocular globe must change over time. It is quite possible to believe that the phenomenon of the ocular globe lengthening is also influenced by the extrinsic ocular musculature, as suggested by Bates (1981/1920).

Numerous studies have been carried out in animals concerning this theory and the effects that retinal defocus has on refraction changes. Schaeffel et al. (1988) and Irving (1991, 1992) proved this by testing chickens with the use of positive and negative lenses. This produces a transitory condition of myopia and hypermetropia. This process results in the ocular globe growing toward the applied plus or minus lens, or in other words, in the direction of compensating refractive errors.

Therefore, the eyes must look through positive lenses (to get a transitory fogging/myopia) to develop a shorter length of the ocular globe axis (thus becoming more positive), thereby counterbalancing the effect induced by the applied positive lens. (The Power Vision System is based on this fact for reducing refractive errors.)

The eyes, treated with the applied negative lenses, demonstrate an increase in the depth of the vitreous chamber. This means that the ocular structure of the eye does in fact change with the applied minus lens. Thus, these eyes develop axial myopia purely as a function of the applied minus lens.

By terminating the stimulation of the lenses at the right

moment, you can prevent myopia from becoming "hypermetropia," a potential consequence of adaptation of the SAID Principle to the focal state imposed by positive lenses (myopic defocus). By using this concept of accommodative balance, we can control the focal state of the eye to meet our distant visual requirements—of maintaining clear distance vision for life. (See the section on Accommodative Balance in Chapter 2.) The stress (due to overaccommodation) creates accommodative hypertonus and, consequently, a condition of transitory defocus (pseudo-myopia) that can become fixed myopia over time.

The opposite of this phenomenon is a kind of defocus induced by a condition of instantaneous and transitory fogging/defocus, which creates the "ground" for changing the refractive conditions until complete, counterbalancing the previous error.

The Importance of Mechanical Forces
for Onset and Development of Myopia

Experimental results show that, in certain circumstances, some mechanical forces are strong enough to arouse ocular globe deformation (typical for axial myopia). Among these mechanical forces are those of ocular muscles and hydraulic pressure, which is caused by too-high intraocular pressure (IOP).

Ocular muscles can make a force that moves the ocular globe; its value is 150 grams (5 ounces) maximum (Robinson, 1964). High IOP level, which is caused by a higher level of focusing and convergence in near vision, increases hydraulic pressure enough to cause ocular globe axial elongation.

Mechanical factors like muscular strength and hydraulic pressure, acting over weakened tissues, become strong enough to set on myopia development. It's important to point out that muscular strength has two components: On one side is active muscular work, together with its voluntary contraction, and on the other side is passive force or resistance, which is caused by different levels of muscular atrophy. Disused or little-used muscles in the situation of high accommodation/convergence (AC/A) and wearing glasses can make for passive muscular resistance. It justifies the extrinsic ocular muscles' work at their highest range of movement (active stretching) in the Power Vision System.

Among mechanical factors suitable to set on myopia development (muscular strength and hydraulic pressure), we should mention also the ciliary muscle, of which chronic contraction can indirectly stimulate the other two mechanisms. If the ciliary muscle is chronically contracted (overaccommodative stress), it causes a focal point shifting (hyperopic defocus; focal point is beyond retina), triggering the intervention of adjusting the focal plane/retina toward that point. This microshifting may cause (with time) ocular globe lengthening and myopia itself.

A vicious circle of action/reaction is set up. It is caused by overaccommodative stress (near-point stress), actually by hyperopic defocus. The action/reaction cycle can be schematized as follows:

- Near target

- Hyperopic defocus (if constant for a long time)

- Chronically contracted ciliary muscle

- Focal plane is trying to be adjusted toward hyperopic focal plane

- Ocular muscles' intervention (due to the previous step)

- Relationship of accommodation/convergence and intraocular pressure increase due to mechanical and hydraulic stress development

- Ocular globe axial elongation and myopia development

Keep in mind: The preceding schematic is only an indicative order regarding the intervention of different forces and mechanisms. Even if interacting in a different way, the result would be the same: a vicious cycle and axial myopia as the final result.

Myopia: Is It Hereditary or Acquired (Environmental)?

Clearing up this question enables us to develop and practice preventive methods, also called "visual reeducation."

There are two different scientific opinions:

1. The first theory (Donders-Helmholtz) states that myopia has heredity as the basic "cause" of nearsightedness.

2. The alternative concept (Helmholtz-dynamic) sees myopia as an acquired error (negative focal status) due to "environmental" causes—actually due to incorrect (bad) use of the eyes. This means wrong or bad use of the eyes in conditions and circumstances that establish a physiologic adaptation, thereby generating negative refractive errors like myopia.

The most convincing logic is the latter opinion (dynamic eye) that myopia is an *acquired defect.* The proof is that most people who have this refractive status were completely healthy at a young age. There are also many scientific studies and facts that back up this assessment.

A study carried out on monkeys (Young, 1971) has proven that the conditions of nearsightedness develop when a hood is used to limit the monkeys' sight. Their eyes, in the laboratory, were forced to view objects at less than 20 inches distance. The scientists found that 75% of monkeys developed myopia within three months.

In addition, the scientists checked the monkeys in an "open" visual environment. Guess what: Virtually no monkeys were nearsighted in this group. Only when they were placed in a laboratory did their focal status change toward nearsightedness (Young, 1965).

One of the most convincing studies on the environmental development of a negative focal status (nearsightedness) was conducted with a large number of Eskimos in Alaska (Young, 1969). The study showed that almost no nearsightedness existed in the grandparents. A small amount existed in the parents, and a large amount developed in the children.

This study was carried out on a sample of 508 people, ages 6 to 88. No myopic error was found among the oldest generation—older than 50 years. Among the younger, fewer than 5% of people aged 41 to 50 were myopic, 23% of people aged 31 to 40, and 43% of those aged 26 to 30. The incidence of myopia among Eskimos aged from 21 to 25 was an astonishing 88%!

The clear explanation of such results lies in the fact that younger generations were gradually exposed to the process of civilization and urbanizing that necessarily put them in such environmental conditions. This condition produced myopia. A further reason was that working and studying at near distances necessarily produced overaccommodative stress.

We should be aware of the importance and prevalence of environmental factors for developing nearsightedness. Let us learn to trust more in the process of natural healing through "ending" the near environment with a plus lens. Enhancing this understanding will allow us to free ourselves from misconceptions that are so rampant about the behavior of the natural eye.

We should terminate the idea that nothing can be done to prevent and reverse nearsightedness. The idea that there is nothing you can do but purchase either expensive negative-lens glasses or contact lenses is a tragic mistake. If we fail to learn this lesson, we will be stuck with being nearsighted for the rest of our lives.

Chapter 2

The Power Vision Test

Verification of Symmetry, Convergence, and Coordination of the Extrinsic Ocular Muscles

The Power Vision System (PVS) is based upon training the ocular muscles in order to correct their lack of strength, flexibility, and coordination. These muscles have the responsibility for accurate control of accommodation and "pointing" of the eyes. The starting point for effective intervention with these types of problems is to determine the nature of these muscular defects. (Lateral and front views of the optical muscles are presented in Figure 2.1a and 2.1b.)

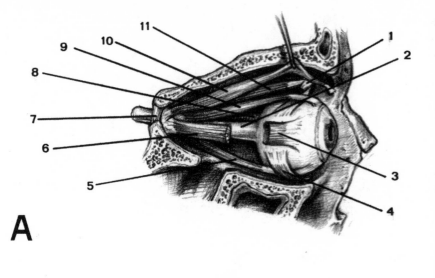

A

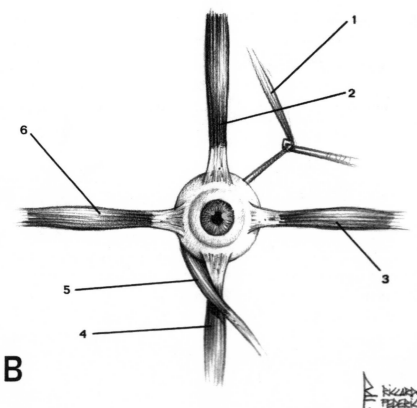

B

Riccardo Federico

Figure 2.1a   *Lateral view of the ocular muscles.*

1. Trochlea

2. Optic nerve

3. Rectus bulbi lateralis muscle (sec.)

4. Obliquus bulbi lateralis muscle

5. Rectus bulbi inferior muscle

6. Rectus bulbi lateralis muscle (sec.)

7. Common tendon ring

8. Rectus bulbi medialis muscle

9. Rectus bulbi superior muscle

10. Levator palpebrae superioris muscle

11. Obliquus bulbi superior muscle

Figure 2.1b   *Front view of the ocular muscles.*

1. Obliquus bulbi superior muscle

2. Rectus bulbi superior muscle

3. Rectus bulbi medialis muscle

4. Rectus bulbi inferior muscle

5. Obliquus bulbi inferior muscle

6. Rectus bulbi lateralis muscle

For other kinds of muscular training, it is necessary to know your own deficiencies (for example, strength, joint mobility, motor coordination, or endurance) to set up *specific* programs of athletic training. This is similar to requirements of other sports disciplines: you determine the training and discipline that you judge are necessary to accomplish a specific result.

This analogy to sports is very suitable for eye training. For the purpose of decreasing myopia, the crucial point is to optimize the "conditional capabilities" of your eyes—through specific exercises—and to learn the "athletic training" of correct focusing. This will be the basis of your own visual conditioning and capabilities.

The Test

Stand in front of a mirror, at about 36 inches distance. The distance you stand from the mirror is the basis of your own focusing capacity. The limit is calculated at the point where you can still see both your pupils clearly. The more myopic you are, the more you must get closer to the mirror in order to see the symmetry and fusion of your eyes.

Position 1

While *constantly* looking at a selected point (for example, the middle of your eyes or at the tip of your nose), lower your chin, keeping your glance fixed at the chosen central point. Maintain your glance and the pupils *at the maximum limit.*

Position 2

While *constantly* looking at a steady point—in the middle of your eyes or the top of your nose—lift your chin up until you reach your limit. In this extreme position, one eye could perform a different convergence from the other, and it might be very hard to maintain convergence in such a position.

Position 3

While looking at a steady point, turn your head to the *left* until the limit is reached where you can still see with both your eyes without hiding one of your pupils behind your nose.

Position 4

While looking at a steady point, turn your head to the *right* until the limit is reached where you can still see both your eyes without hiding one of your eyes with your nose. The same exercise is to be repeated in the other four directions of your visual field.

Position 5

While looking at a steady point, incline your glance down toward your *right* as far as you can.

Position 6

Looking at a steady point, incline your glance down toward the *left* as far as you can.

Position 7

While looking at a steady point, incline your glance up toward the *right* as far as you can.

Position 8

While looking at a steady point, incline your glance up toward the *left* as far as you can.

It will be hard to maintain the perfect convergence in these extreme positions, so you might have double vision. This phenomenon will become more apparent in certain positions.

These errors in convergence demonstrate a flexibility defect as well as the incapability of maintaining a long fixed glance in such positions. This action demonstrates a strength defect of the *agonist* muscles (those muscles that are resisted or counteracted by another muscle, the *antagonist*), and consequently a coordination error.

Weak muscles, with defects in muscular symmetry and improper convergence in one or more directions of the visual fields, lead to inexact accommodation and adjustment, jeopardizing visual functioning. It is very hard, and perhaps impossible, to "point" to an object and make its image fall on the central fovea—the most sensitive retinal portion for accurate focus—in these conditions of muscular imbalance and asymmetry.

The Power Vision System is aimed at improving the "athletic" capabilities of the eyes *gradually* and *specifically* with valid and evident improvements. Results will be gradually achieved—restoring the eye's extrinsic muscles' symmetry, strengthening them, and increasing their flexibility. All this great work is carried out using the physiologic SAID Principle (Specific Adaptation to the Imposed Demand) through the wise use of lenses with gradations opposite to the corrective one—positive lenses for nearsighted and negative lenses for farsighted people—together with the CRB (Contraction/Relaxation/Blinking) eye movements (explained more fully in Chapter 5).

Muscular Rehabilitation

Striated or "voluntary" muscles work as pairs.

Every muscle is both agonist and antagonist; it depends on which movements are involved (that is, in arm flexion the agonist muscle is the biceps, and the antagonist is the triceps muscle. In arm extension, the agonist is the triceps and the antagonist the biceps.) Due to the stretch reflex called "reciprocal innervation," when the agonist contracts, the antagonist *relaxes*. This stretch reflex helps the muscle to lengthen and helps coordination for the best execution. In the eye muscle, the active static stretching exercises help relax the antagonist muscle and develop strength in the agonist.

The best eye stretching exercise is the "rotation from a fixed point" test described previously, because it permits the feedback of perfect coordination. For *best* results, once some muscular imbalance in coordination is found (when the vision doubles in extreme positions of the visual field), one must continue in those positions searching for ocular fusion, searching to *relax* the eye muscle in those extreme positions (standing in front of the mirror, rotate the head, searching for the field of double vision, and try to relax, searching for ocular fusion). After some time you eventually will experience clearer vision and improved acuity.

This exercise will ensure the best and fastest results because it greatly improves the muscular performance of the eye muscle (best central fixation and coordination) in those visual fields where it is most needed. The "specificity" of the visual range where the stretching is applied in this exercise is the reason for its efficacy.

The first phase of implementing functional rehabilitation will produce a gradual improvement in your focusing capacity. It includes muscular training, which occurs because the agonist and antagonistic muscles are strengthened.

This phase acts on their properties (strength, flexibility, and coordination) gradually. Working with this muscular group of the six extrinsic eye muscles restores their coordination. It increases the eye's "central fixation" ability and improves the eye's dynamic (*saccadic*) movements. The "plasticity" of the striated muscles has been established by the research carried out in monkeys by A. B. Scott in 1994.

This research was aimed at defining whether the extraocular muscular system of the monkeys had the capacity of adapting (that is, the feature of "plasticity"). The research determined that the monkeys' extrinsic muscles—being held in the state of lengthening through sutures—lengthen at 18%, 25%, and 33%. Obviously, in the case of PVS, muscular rehabilitation and the restoration of extrinsic eye muscle functioning isn't achieved by suturing the muscles. It is achieved through the systematic work of ocular stretching at the maximum ranges of the ocular field.

Two Fundamental Factors

The two fundamental factors of ocular stretching are (1) strength increase and (2) training load increase or a gradual intensity increase.

Strength Increase

Since we are working toward a strength increase of the eye's extrinsic muscles—which are of the striated type—the muscles are subject to the very same rules as any other striated bodily muscle (calf, triceps). The strength of these muscles depends on their capacity of working—shifting a load—over a certain period of time. Similar to strength exercises such as bodybuilding, the muscles carry out dynamic contractions—eccentric and concentric types—in which the trained muscle varies its length to the applied load. An example would be working with a barbell.

When increasing the strength of the eye's extrinsic muscles, the contractions are of the isometric type, where the resistance is steady and exists even without movement of the visible load. Obviously it is impossible to get a barbell or physical load onto the ocular muscle. In such cases, the resistance is given by the antagonistic muscle, which opposes the movement.

For example, let us review one of your muscular work movements—the one of fixing at a point at the extreme left part of the visual field on a horizontal level. In this movement, the strength of the agonist muscles—musculus rectus on the left side—will increase, and the flexibility of the antagonistic muscles—musculus rectus on the right side—will improve. In the opposite movement—when you fix at the extreme right part of the visual field on a horizontal level—the situation will be different. The strength of the musculi recti, which is agonist in this movement, will increase, and the lengthening capacity of the musculi recti on the left side (antagonistic muscles in this case) will be increased.

Doing these exercises in all sections of the visual field—schematized in eight positions—points to where the imbalance is more evident. Your eyes' performance is necessarily being gradually improved through this muscular rehabilitation.

The contraction "intensity" factor is the fundamental concept for such rehabilitative work and must be pondered carefully to achieve efficient training stimulus and to generate the required muscular tissue adaptation. A small training stimuli, like very weak contractions, leads to little or no results. However, a well-measured contraction intensity leads to stimulus optimizing, with additional overcompensation. This means muscle adaptation to the stimulus—better muscular performance, and consequently more accurate "pointing."

You can analyze an overcompensation graph—meant as a performance/functional capacity increase of an organ or system of organs—usually used to highlight improvement of sports performance capacities. Muscular work—in this case, doing the work of fixing at extreme parts of the visual field—leads to an initial drop of the trained muscle's efficiency. In the case of ocular muscle training, this phase is characterized by a transient and physiological drop in focusing capacity.

After a suitable recovery time, the muscle both overcompensates—becomes used to the training load given by the exercise

—and, as a physiological consequence, develops better properties—strength, flexibility, and resistance. As for the extrinsic ocular muscles, the result will be better coordination and "pointing"
of the eyes. These muscles are responsible for saccadic movements
and central focusing. Proper tone of these muscles is essential for
accurate, clear vision.

Intensity Evaluation in Ocular Exercises

How can we calculate load intensity in ocular isometric exercises—fixing the borders of the visual field—if we cannot vary
and/or measure it "by sight"? We do this in ordinary strength
exercises when we change the weight on a barbell. We can compare it to the forms of isometric strength increases by any striated
bodily muscle.

That is the relationship between contraction duration and the
range of movement—but in the case of the eyes, the range of
the lever can't be taken into account because the length of the
limbs does not exist. The person who has organic visual problems—cataracts, glaucoma, and/or retinal detachment—should
not do these exercises.

Optimal Intensity

To achieve intense contraction—efficient stimulus—focusing is
maintained at an extreme level as long as possible, until you feel
a slight muscular tiredness. However, your contraction intensity should be evaluated by an optometrist who understands the
concepts of the Power Vision System. Therefore, the opinion of
a physician or a specialist is advisable.

Training Load Increase or a Gradual Intensity Increase

It is very important to adjust the stimulus to your new visual
capacities from time to time so as to maintain the stimulus

intensity efficiently and to be able to bring about visual system adaptation.

Such training load variation in the ocular stretching exercises can be done by increasing the number and the wideness of ocular rotations as well as the duration of maintaining each position at the extreme point of the visual field (in such cases, the more the speed is decreasing, the more the contraction intensity is increasing).

The relationship of lens to reading distance should be gradually increased in the exercises with lenses (positive for nearsighted/ myopic people). Once you are able to read at an arm's length distance with +1 diopter positive lenses, you should proceed to the +1.50 or +2.0 lens, reading at the distance where you have a slightly blurred vision by trying to focus the text doing CRB movements. In the case of low myopia—when wearing the plus lenses indoors at home or at the office—so as to reduce environmental near-point stress, you should slightly increase the "leisure" lens-induced blur. Slightly myopic or nearly emmetropic people should wear positive lenses at home or at the office. In the case of moderate to high myopia, it is not necessary to wear positive training lenses at home or at the office. It will be enough to wear lenses slightly weaker than the prescribed ones for close work.

If you don't carry out gradual training load increasing, you will be confined within the limits of the already reached adaptation of your visual system to that kind of stimulus (rotation intensity, the power of training lenses) and, consequently, within the achieved improvements.

Wherever you are, *always* respect safety rules. If I work in an airport control tower, or if I am a pilot or bus driver where I am required to have perfect sight, I'll avoid "myopizing" my eyes even for therapeutic reasons. Therefore, I'll wear *full* correction lenses for my refractive error.

The same rules apply to personal and collective safety and must be respected. You take complete responsibility for your own actions. Neither the optometrist nor specialist can be blamed for anything under this circumstance.

Therapeutic Validity of Ocular Stretching: Relationship of Length to Muscular Tension

Active and passive work on oculomotor muscles through active stretching finds its therapeutic validity in the physiological foundation of the relationship of length to muscular tension.

Any imbalance causes lower efficiency in "pointing" movable targets, lower and imprecise focusing capability on central fovea (central fixation), as well as lower saccadic vibration capability (because of slow and "dulled" muscles). The quality of ocular muscles' work and of all the striated muscles in general depends on harmonious interaction between agonist and antagonistic muscles in a certain movement. Any strength and flexibility imbalance causes a lower capability of working and moving, because of a lower level of active contracting and a higher level of passive resistance created by little-used muscles.

As you can see in Figure 2.2, optimal muscular movement, or its optimal active working (contracting), can be performed when the muscle is in optimal length range. A chronically contracted muscle or, conversely, a too-stretched muscle, can't perform its function of action/reaction/movement optimally. Analyzing this problem thoroughly, we find that there are two microfilaments that are fundamental components of a muscle: actin and myosin. Muscular contracting comes from these two components sliding one over the other. Stretching happens the opposite way: when the level of superposition between actin and myosin gradually decreases. Opposite to contraction, muscular stretching itself happens in a "passive" way: In the case of ocular muscles, where gravitation can't act, stretching happens passively, thanks to the agonist muscle.

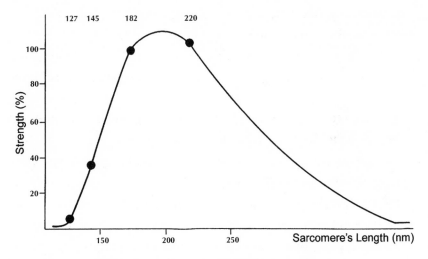

Figure 2.2   Relationship of muscular length to tension.

When all the range of the movement isn't completely used (as happens when limited visual ranges are used due to the frame of the glasses), the muscular capability of active contracting becomes lower, as does muscular elasticity itself, affecting fundamental factors for optimal vision like the capability of pointing, central fixation (centralization), and saccadic movements. If ocular stretching is performed *symmetrically* and within the extreme range of the visual field, it preserves and restores the optimal relationship between length and muscular tension, which is very important for correct, clear, distinct vision.

Relationship between Focusing and Visual Field Width

We can use the SAID Principle here. The eye adapts to the environmentally imposed requests.

As has already been discussed, there is a close relationship between the development of myopia and prolonged close work. In studies carried out on pigeons, researchers discovered a different refractive capacity in different sections of the visual field (Catania, 1964; Millodot & Blough, 1971; Nye, 1973). The pigeons had normal sight when their refractive state was measured when their eye was measured along its own axis, on the frontal level. The more the pupil axis got closer to the lower visual field, the more myopia was increased (Fitzke et al., 1985).

This interesting result shows that the visual system can selectively adapt to its environment, since the bird must both focus on near objects for feeding and at the same time have a correct alignment of the upper parts of its visual field to see birds of prey.

It is important to keep in mind that the variability of such refractive conditions is *not* steady within a species. The animal's eye adapted to its visual environment (see Miles & Wallman, 1990).

The Reason Why Wearing Glasses Prevents Recovery

The eye adapts its focal status to the near visual field. When this happens, a minus lens is prescribed. This lens has a negative effect on the human eye. The minus lens produces an overaccommodative effect. Further, the minus-lens glasses limit normal range of eye movement. Wearing any pair of glasses necessarily limits motion. The eyes hardly ever have room because of the limits imposed by the frame (see Figure 2.3). Such restriction of eye-movement range over time leads to the extrinsic ocular muscles adapting to the range of motion imposed by the frame of the glasses.

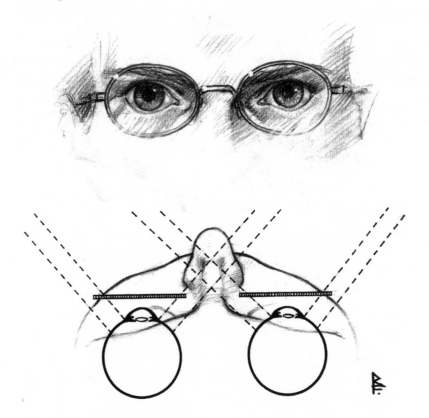

Figure 2.3   Limited visual range.

The frame of the glasses hinders and limits the entire eye movement with the consequent decrease of the extraocular muscles' working range.

As a result there is an *in pejus* (negative) adaptation by the extrinsic muscles' elastic capacities. A further consequence is the loss of coordination and quality of saccadic movements. In such a "cage," the eye's visual field is imprisoned; this leads to eyestrain and stiffness—with further development of myopia.

These facts were emphasized by Dr. William H. Bates (1881–1920), the father and pioneer of visual rehabilitation. He pointed out that the stiffness and steadiness of the gaze, as well as muscular tension, are the principal causes for defective sight.

Just remember that when a striated muscle is being subjected to a decrease in its normal range of movement, it gradually develops decreased flexibility and coordination. In the case of the extrinsic eye muscles, their flexibility is directly correlated with their coordinating capabilities and is part of their fundamental capability.

How the Power Vision System Acts on the Visual Field

The Power Vision System exercises the ocular muscles through ocular rotations—with some variations—at the maximum range of ocular movement.

These motions rehabilitate and prevent the elastic ocular capabilities of the visual field from narrowing. This narrowing occurs because of the habitual wearing of glasses. PVS restores these necessary capabilities of the natural eye—like strength and flexibility—needed for optimal saccadic movement and clear vision.

Retinal Defocus: Active Emmetropization and SAID Principle

Active emmetropization is a phenomenon in which the eye adjusts its focal status to its environment. The process is seen in the eye's tendency to bring its refractive state closer to zero—defined as *emmetropic* or clear sight. This phenomenon demonstrates the natural eye's capacity of changing its refractive power toward the applied visual environment. (The word *emmetropia* means a focal state of exactly zero. Most eyes with 20/20 vision have a focal status of zero to +1.5 diopters [Hayden, 1941]).

The effect of this emmetropization process is clear as it applies to humans. Proper modification of the near environment with a plus lens will help the natural eye emmetropize in a positive direction—thus clearing distance vision.

A slightly nearsighted person who does not wear his minus-lens glasses for some time can notice an adaptation of his focusing capacity in a positive direction. This is a consequence of the active emmetropization stimulus. Not wearing the glasses reduces the hyperopic defocus that is caused by traditional negative optical correction (allowing a certain margin for this emmetropization process to work properly. I grant that gradual emmetropization of refractive error is a slow process. For this reason it is necessary to back up the adaptation of the eye to the lenses through suitable and gradual use of the defocus state).

Active Emmetropization in Animals

The phenomenon of active emmetropization has been noticed for some time in experiments with animals. These experiments demonstrate a recovery from nearsighted (nonzero) refractive states. The eye has the ability of compensating for lens-driven retinal defocus.

The first evidence for active emmetropization—the eye's response to its visual environment—following an induced myopic state was identified in chickens (Wallman & Adams, 1987; Norton, 1990; McBrien & Norton, 1992). The study carried out on the monkeys reported that the primate eye demonstrated a recovery from retinal defocus induced by contact lenses that were experimentally used on these animals (Smith et al., 1994). The studies in monkeys, chickens, and guinea pigs show an adaptation of the visual system—active emmetropization to the visual environment—in response to lens-driven refractive errors.

The effect of applying an external negative lens produced a net negative change in focal status of the eye. The effect of applying an external positive lens produced a net positive change in focal status of the eye. This is because of the eye's ability to change its length proportional to the applied plus or minus lens, that is, the dynamic and innate emmetropization process. The test demonstrates that the ocular refractive state can be changed suitably by correct application of the correct lens for recovery and prevention.

A mildly myopic person, subjected to certain stimuli—myopic defocus led by positive lenses or undercorrections—will with time decrease his refractive error. If this process is initiated before the minus lens is used, the eye's focal status can potentially be cleared back to normal (emmetropia). The opposite concept works as well. A hyperopic person, subject to minus-lens hyperopic defocus, can decrease his positive refractive error and get close to an emmetropic state. (I can personally testify to, and prove—apart from clear scientific results—the success of this process in humans, specifically concerning recovery from myopia, since I worked myself out of it over a period of ten years.)

The phenomenon of active emmetropization is an expression of the SAID Principle, meaning that the eye has bidirectional control. This compensating ability acts in response to the use of either positive or negative lenses (myopic or hyperopic defocus).

Retinal Defocus and Refractive Change

The theory of accommodation behavior suggests that after
some time retinal position is changed to better
coincide with focal point of the lens-retina system.
—Theodore Grosvenor and David A. Goss,
Clinical Management of Myopia

Current studies carried out on animals suggest that refractive development and, therefore, the refractive state are modulated by the accommodation status and the clarity of focus of retinal image. Defocus of the retinal image with minus lenses causes an acceleration and enlargement of the vitreous chamber. This results in myopia. The plus lenses cause a slowing of the axial elongation of the eye, allowing for the prevention of nearsightedness (Schaeffel et al., 1988; Schaeffel & Howland, 1991; Irving, 1991; Grosvenor & Goss, 1999, p. 54).

Experiments on Retinal Defocus Using Primates

The possibility of altering refractive development by inducing retinal defocus (change) was first studied by Hung et al. in 1995, using young monkeys. The study proved that the focal status of Rhesus monkeys was profoundly changed by the forced wearing of a plus or minus lens.

The monkeys wore helmets so the lens could be kept in place. The left eye was used as the control and the right eye had variously a +6, +3, 0, −3, and −6 diopter lens applied. The monkeys were from 21 to 32 days old at the start of the test to confirm the eye's dynamic response to these applied lenses. The test continued for 72 to 113 days.

At the end of the experiment the refractive change was measured with retinoscopy. The initial focal states of the monkeys were from 2 to 8 diopters. (With respect to the starting focal status, the left eye is almost always very close to the right eye, with a "spread" of about 0.5 diopters.)

The result of this test demonstrated that the right eye followed the applied lens. If the lens was plus, the right eye went more plus (moved in a hyperopic direction). If the applied lens was minus, the focal status moved in a negative direction (that is, moved in a "nearsighted" direction).

This test demonstrated that the natural eye uses its environment or the applied lens to control its long-term focal status. According to the theory of accommodative balance, if the treatment had been stopped at the right moment, the emmetropic state would have been achieved without developing hyperopia. So it is obvious that the refractive state is influenced by the defocus on the retina and that you can voluntarily control your refractive status by modifying your environment, thereby preventing a negative focal status from developing.

PVS provides a system enabling a gradual decrease of refractive errors toward 20/20 vision. It takes its basis from the connection between the development of myopia and near-work, as well as from the eye's ability to react to induced change in the visual environment. Many studies—carried out in humans and animals—clearly show how the visual system, because of its focusing capacity, changes its focal status as the environment is changed.

There's a close relationship between the development of myopia and environmentally induced refractive conditions. This is the case when working indoors. The eye can't adjust to longer focusing distances, so the accommodation system "steers" the eye into nearsightedness.

Such facts are clearly demonstrated in humans. By analyzing this relationship (myopia development by environmentally induced near-point stress/refractive stress), we can confirm different myopic development depending on work and environmentally induced near-point stress (overaccommodation). On the basis of this correlation between the refractive state changes and environmentally induced change, we can see the possibilities for acting on the *causes* of the problem—the defocused state. Such knowledge allows us not only to prevent myopia from developing but to also act voluntarily to decrease it.

Your refractive state can be consciously manipulated by you. This depends on the kind of refractive error you have (nearsightedness or farsightedness) providing a suitable stimulus. This applied lens is aimed at the visual system's ability to adapt, consequently helping restore your distance vision to normal.

Such an aim can be achieved through retinal defocus: in the case of nearsightedness, to decrease myopic functional errors using positive lenses or undercorrections; for hyperopic retinal defocus, to decrease hyperopic refractive errors by using a negative lens.

Myopic Defocus

Myopic defocus occurs when the accommodative stimulus exceeds the individual's amplitude of accommodation by approximately 1 to 2 diopters, producing increased amounts of underaccommodation and consequent retinal image defocus. Beyond this point, the accommodative response becomes progressively smaller and gradually shifts toward the tonic accommodative level (Ong & Ciuffreda, 1997). (See Figures 2.4, 2.5, 2.6.)

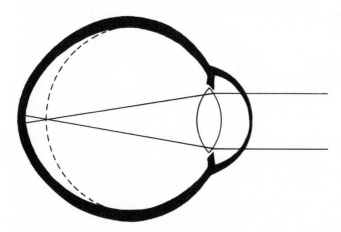

Figure 2.4   Myopic eye.

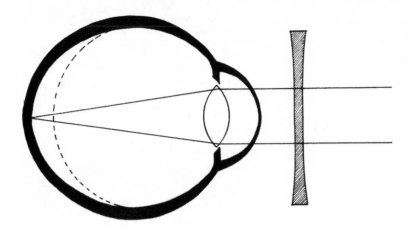

Figure 2.5　Optical correction for myopic eye with a concave lens (–).

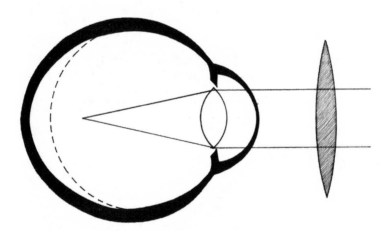

*Figure 2.6　Myopic defocus induced by a convex lens (+) on
myopic eye.*

Hyperopic Defocus

If the dioptric stimulus is progressively positioned beyond optical
infinity (possible only with optical systems), the accommodative
response gradually shifts (relative to the response at optical infin-

ity) slightly higher toward the tonic accommodative level (Ong & Ciuffreda, 1997). (See Figures 2.7–2.11.)

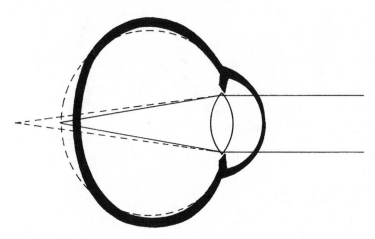

Figure 2.7   Hyperopic eye.

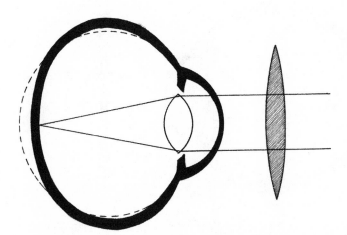

Figure 2.8   Optical correction of the hyperopic eye with a convex lens (+).

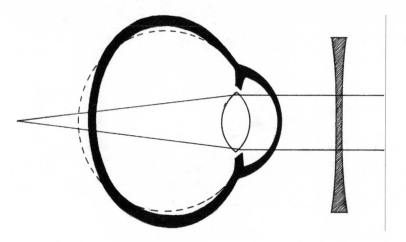

Figure 2.9   Hyperopic defocus by concave lens (–) on hyperopic eye.

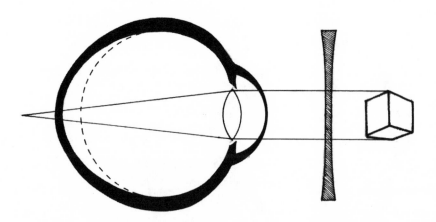

Figure 2.10   Hyperopic defocus by convex lens (–) on myopic eye.

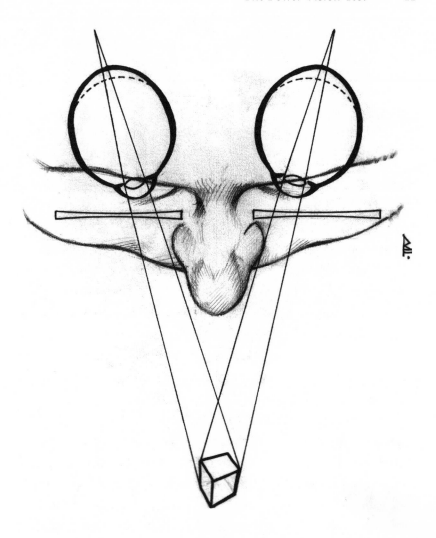

Figure 2.11 Hyperopic defocus induced by the use of negative (concave) lenses—reproduces the effect of near vision on the eyes focal status. In addition, convergence acts as a further myopic impulse.

In short:

- Defocus is of the myopic type when using positive lenses or undercorrections. This is because the focal point of ocular imagery is shifted in front of the retina.

- Defocus is of the hyperopic type when, using negative lenses, the focal point of ocular imagery is shifted behind the retina.

Such retinal defocus stimuli are artificially produced in the Power Vision System by using lenses or undercorrections. In this case, both the adaptation and the refractive visual error counterbalancing are found through the suitable state of defocus/fogging.

The retinal defocus state also occurs under normal conditions when we fix on a distant object and then immediately turn our glance to a near object—instantaneously, and before starting the accommodative response, the focus is behind the retina. When the accommodative response is less than the dioptric stimulus (as controlled suitably with lenses), a certain level of hyperopic defocus will remain (Wildsoet, 1998, p. 35).

This stimulation leads to the adaptation of the eye's refractive capability and consequently its focusing—compensating for the initial refractive error. Such a system of retinal defocus, being prolonged over time, allowed me to decrease my myopia gradually, by 2 diopters in each eye. The complete defocus state, induced by lenses, acts as an overaccommodative balance, thereby providing the rationale for a functional adaptation of the focusing system.

Unsuitable use of defocus, as occurs with current optical "corrections" (hyperopic defocus for nearsighted people through negative lenses, and myopic defocus for farsighted people through positive lenses) tends to worsen visual errors, thus "spoiling" the natural eye's refractive capabilities. Medina and Fariza (1993) reasoned that the traditional correction of myopia with negative lenses inserts an initial error that causes hyperopic defocus and accelerates nearsightedness progression (that is, worsening). How many pairs of glasses have you changed up to now, increasing the dioptric power of the lenses each time, following this traditional method of correction?

To make this concept completely clear—even to the nonspecialist reader—let me say this: a treadmill carrying a still person (one who was not moving his legs) from one side to the other would hardly ever stimulate the person's locomotion and walking. Running or walking with increasingly heavier ballast, on the contrary, stimulates one's physiological abilities to a large degree.

What hinders might strengthen, what helps might destroy, bringing about an undesired adaptation of a physiological system. Such a principle explains the behavior of most physiological systems. A suitable optical stimulus creates the adaptation of the focusing system to the lens as part of the SAID Principle.

The effect of lenses on focal adjustment can be found in many scientific works, such as Smith (1998). Retinal defocus induced by near-work and, if worsened by hyperopic defocus (induced by negative lenses for myopia), will in time lead to axial myopia, that is, eyeball lengthening. (See Smith & Hung, 1995; Raviola & Wiesel, 1985; Wallman, 1993).

Accommodative Balance

The eye's refractive capacity is influenced by environmental factors—as when the observed object is near. Refractive capacity is affected by emotional factors; our mood can affect our wish to see the observed object. For instance, a severe glance by someone in authority, repeated many times, can cause us to withdraw from the world into a state of comfortable blur, that is, into our "own world." The eye is a living and vibrant organ, and its refractive status is the sum of all the stimuli that impinge on it.

Your ocular status is characterized by what I define as *accommodative balance*. Your focal status is the result of all physical and mental stimuli, that is, your environment. These stimuli are imposed on your eyes whether you like it or not. The major stimulus here is overaccommodative stress, induced by near-work. Improvement would be accommodative relaxation, induced by looking at distance, light, and improving the working range of ocular muscles. It is extremely important to understand this concept so as to reduce refractive errors—since you must count on this mechanism to change your refractive state in a positive direction.

Your refractive status is maintained if there is a balance between myopic and hyperopic stimuli (see Figure 2.12). For instance, if myopic stimuli (close work) overcome the hyperopic (distant viewing), this will eventually produce a refractive change toward myopia. Such a phenomenon is nothing else but the reaction and adaptation of a visual system to the applied stimuli—and that is the specific expression of the SAID Principle.

Figure 2.12   Accommodative balance, or the eye in a state of equilibrium.

[left] Visual stimuli at near distance

[right] Visual stimuli at far distance

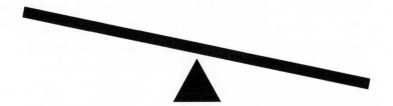

Figure 2.13   The prevalence of near vision stimuli causes a change of accommodative balance toward myopia.

[left] Visual stimuli at far distance

[right] Visual stimuli at near distance

[right] Stress of the nervous system

Fundamental characteristics required to generate a change in someone's refractive capacity include:

- Induction of a suitable kind of stimulus (either myopic or hyperopic, depending on the initial functional refractive error)
- Induction of enough intense stimulus or defocus (either too much or too little intense stimuli do not create an adaptation)
- The time of exposure to stimuli (the quantity of time being exposed to defocus must be so great as to induce a transient change of your refractive state)

Such exposure tends to transiently change the accommodative balance with time, causing steadier and steadier changes and becoming a part of one's normal refractive capabilities. A myopic person, trained with myopic defocus on a regular basis, little by little will get closer to the emmetropic state, intervening over his accommodative balance.

Denying the theory of accommodative balance would mean denying the capacity of all the organs and physiological systems to adapt or modify themselves to various induced stimuli. It would mean denying the physiological principle of Specific Adaptation to the Imposed Demand. The heart gets used to the stimuli that are induced in aerobic training. The skin undergoes adaptation to temperature and light rays. The muscles get used to the induced load. There are countless examples of stimulation that impinge on a living organism.

So—why should the eyes and their refractive state be different? One's refractive status changes in relation to environmentally induced stimuli. Or this change is willingly caused and led by a specific visual training. By using plus lenses or undercorrections suitably, you can change your visual environment. The result will be a gradual adaptation of your refractive status in a positive direction and a resultant clearing of your distance vision.

Prevention and Treatment of Myopia
with Positive Lenses or Undercorrections

It is documented by scientific experimentation and in technical publications that your refractive state is regulated by the diopter power of your visual environment. This includes both the quality and kind of refractive stimuli that impinge on your eyes. Therefore, the eye and its refractive capability to change are influenced by accidental stimuli (like overaccommodative stress induced by near-work) or by willingly and artificially induced stimuli designed to cause either adaptation or compensation for the induced defocus.

The experiments carried out on animals are very significant (Hung et al., 1995; Schaeffel, 1988; Siegwart & Norton, 1993; McFadden & Wallman, 1995). In these studies, lenses were used to induce specific adaptations of animals' (chickens' and Guinea pigs') refractive state. The result was that the eyes adapted themselves toward myopia, using negative lenses that were causing hyperopic defocus and axial elongation of the eyeball. This "adaptation effect" is the unfortunate result of using the improper optical correction.

Let me repeat: Myopia, when corrected with negative lenses, results in myopia worsening. This is because of increasing overaccommodative stress and inducing hyperopic defocus, which in time sets up the stimulus for axial elongation of the eye (see Medina & Fariza, 1993). Conversely, the wise use of positive lenses or undercorrections, generating transient, artificially induced myopia, causes a myopic retinal defocus. This is a stimulus that compensates for the initial error. In this case the eye is "pushed" to compensate for the initial error so as to restore the optimal refractive state (see Smith, 1998).

All this is a direct expression of the SAID Principle: a specific stimuli leads to a specific adaptation. In this case the result worsens the initial refractive error.

Birnbaum and many other clinicians (Birnbaum, 1988, p. 169) state that the use of positive lenses on the threshold of myopia could prevent nearsightedness in the first place. There are quite a few optometrists who have stated this concept over the past century. The reason for using a preventive lens is to modify your visual environment so as to mitigate or completely remove all the near stimuli. Doing so will lead to a reduction of accommodative stress. And, of course, accommodation stress is recognized as the cause of the gradual development of myopia.

Most existing scientific studies on the use of positive lenses for preventing and reducing myopia were conducted using bifocal lenses. The lower part of the lens was positive (to oppose the effects of overaccommodative stress) and the upper part had either no lens (*plano*) or had a reduced-power negative lens.

Roberts and Banfort (1967) found that the use of bifocal lenses brings about significant reduction in the rate of development of refractive errors. The downward rate developed at –0.31 diopter per year for the test group using a plus lens (bifocal) compared with a rate of –0.41 diopter per year for the control group using the regular minus lens.

The strongest success in preventing negative movement into myopia was conducted by Kenneth Oakley and Francis Young in 1975. In the lower part of the bifocal lenses they used +1.50 diopters, and the upper part of the lens was undercorrected by 0.5 diopters. Oakley and Young determined that the overall average increase of myopic error was –0.02 diopter per year for the bifocal group. The "standard prescription" group continued into myopia at a rate of –0.53 diopter per year. The clear success of this study was attributed to the fact that a sufficiently strong plus lens was used. The "students" were motivated to follow the desired protocol of Francis Young. They were given a strong plus for all close work and a weaker plus for distant viewing.

Many scientific studies confirm the effects of retinal defocus on the refractive state. Each organ adapts to the induced specific stimulation, and the eyes and their refractive capacity are not an exception. The use of gradual myopic defocus (induced by a positive lens or undercorrections) leads toward regressing and gradual compensating for the initial error. The expression "The functioning makes the organ" is very often used in medicine. The expression means, "Each stimulation produces a physiological adaptation."

The Blur-Driven Accommodation Principle

Blurred retinal image requires accommodative innervating
which is aimed at modifying the dioptric power of a crystalline

lens in order to optimize adjustment and thereby achieve clear vision. Retina signals a "focusing error," and this perception sets up a stimulus to modify the innervating "signal" which controls the crystalline lens. That is when the focusing error is canceled and the modifying stimulus stops.
—Gian Paolo Paliaga, *I vizi di refrazione*

This stimulus causes focusing adaptation and optimization and is completely opposite to optical correction with corrective lenses. A focusing stimulus, used *gradually*, generates a natural adaptation of the visual organs and their focusing capacity: it leads to a regression of functional visual errors.

The secret of getting back to 6/6 (20/20, in English units) eyesight—or to decrease your present dioptric prescription—is to use this principle of consistent effort. This means *increasing* the focusing distance *gradually*, so that you recognize the necessity of using a stronger plus lens or undercorrections as you see your distance vision improving.

The Solution for Functional Visual Errors, or Developing an Understanding of Using a Lens to Clear Your Distance Vision

The eye's focusing power depends on several stimuli, including:

- Psychological or physiological conditions (stress, fear)
- Mental and physical tension
- The visual environment
- Artificially induced refractive conditions caused by contact lenses and glasses

Practical and Illustrative Use of the SAID Principle for Improving Sight

A slightly myopic person who trains with a plus lens or undercorrections while reading a book or the newspaper must always discipline himself to read at the "blur point." That is, he must push the reading material *away* from his eyes to the point of "just blurred." This creates a training load for the focusing system. It is as if we trained the extrinsic ocular and the ciliary muscles using a stronger and stronger applied load.

In this case, the load is part of both your reading distance *and* the power of training lenses. Once the focusing system gets used to that load—which is the relationship between dioptric power of the eye and the training distance—it is necessary to increase the load in order to clear your vision further. If this is not done, the stimulus will not continue to have the desired training effect.

This phenomenon, which induces a training accommodative stimulus (for better adjustment with the consequent functional refractive error decrease), is called "fogging," or "blur-driven accommodation"; the eye is voluntarily led to the state of slight fogging so as to be stimulated for focusing. It is *very important* to measure the training stimulus.

With this kind of system, which leads into a slightly burred state (so the letters of the observed text can be hardly distinguished), the eye's refractive state can be modified automatically and gradually so as to bring "focus" back on the retina, or at least, as close as possible. It means that a myopic person, whose focal point is in front of the retina, must shift it to nearer the retina, consequently optimizing focusing. For hyperopic people, whose focal point is behind the retina, the principle works well when used in the opposite direction (negative lenses at the shortest possible distance).

The Importance of Measuring Out
the Light Blur-Driven Training Stimulus

The load or the training stimulus imposed on the eye's focusing capacity must be efficient; that means neither too excessive nor too little. The best training effect is achieved by having minimum fogging, when the letters or the object you are focusing on are slightly out of focus.

Excessive fogging may cause the opposite negative effect, worsening either myopia or hyperopia. The reason might be that in the case of an excessive stimulus, focusing becomes impossible, without even having a try at all.

Chapter 3

My Own Experience in Clearing My Distance Vision

When using the plus lens, my eyesight was getting better and my eyes were approaching normal vision. It was, however, harder and harder to achieve improvements, despite the fact that I was doing ocular stretching and training using "reading" glasses.

While doing this work on recovery, I was diagnosed with 0.50 diopter of myopia in each eye. I had reached the point of reading through positive lenses of +4 diopters (D) with artificial light. I could read in sunlight using +6 diopter lenses. Despite my hard work, my improvements were very slow. It was as if the last traces of my myopia didn't want to let me go—so that I could free and release my eyes.

I often noticed a very interesting fact. The morning after I had been up late, I would notice that my sight was apparently clearer as I went to the office. I didn't understand this. I thought that a short period of sleep would mean that the nervous system had less time to "recover." This system rules homeostasis and consequently is responsible for your well-being. In most cases, physical and mental weariness worsens focusing capability. My own case seemed to be an exception to the rule.

I started wearing a low-power positive lens—not only while training and reading, but also indoors, at home, and at the office. Since I was myopic, I was wearing my positive lenses and needed them to create a blur-driven stimulus to let my eyes get used to it. The result was an increase in their acuity, reducing and eliminating overaccommodative, near-point stress. Even after a night at home working, I would notice better visual acuity in the morning.

I finally understood why. Overaccommodative stress caused by near-work has increased in our society—living and working indoors—so that you hardly glance toward far distance. Environmental factors do indeed contribute to the development and worsening of myopia. Knowing this, we can take the necessary steps to reduce and completely eliminate the indoor stress.

The people whose myopia is very high will find an advantage in *not* wearing glasses indoors and at safe places (like at home), or at most, if their myopia is very high, it would be better to wear lower-power lenses. In the case of low myopia, not wearing lenses indoors won't be enough to decrease the negative state of the overaccommodation condition, but such people should wear "leisure" lenses (positive lenses), which create slightly blurred vision.

In my case, when my myopia decreased at 0.50 D, I was wearing positive lenses +1.00 D at work, and +2.00 D lenses at home (where I felt safe). These elements are personal and approximate: concerning any level of myopia, the precise protocol to learn the right dioptric power of indoor lenses doesn't exist presently.

Everyone, being sensible, should create such slightly blurred vision when indoors, so as not to overload the visual system with excessive near-work. The stimulus (blurred vision) shouldn't ever be excessive, so that it overcomes the suitable level for creating a focusing system adaptation. In the opposite case, if the eye becomes too myopic with positive lenses (even transitory), it is likely to give up trying to focus on the objects and environment, considering it an impossible task.

My visual acuity after a night out was due to the fact that my nervous system wasn't subjected to overaccommodative/near-point stress or the "indoors" stress when I was at home. To avoid this problem I started wearing "leisure" lenses at home and at the office.

Keep in mind: Such positive "leisure" lenses should be worn only when the place or environment and your job don't require full optical correction for safety reasons, common sense, or as prescribed by the law. This indication works well also for the use of undercorrection lenses for nearsightedness with high myopia and in all cases of myopic defocus.

Retinal Defocus Progression: Necessity and Importance

Retinal defocus progression is the fundamental factor to take into account so as to obtain gradual improvement. To achieve improvements, it is necessary to gradually increase the optically induced blur once the visual system is adapted to the relationship between reading distance and training lens power. The same concept works well for hyperopia, but is used in the opposite way: reading distance is to be shortened gradually, using stronger and stronger negative lenses.

I have learned all of this from my personal experience. For more than a year I was imprisoned in a refractive state of –0.50 D in each eye. Even though I was reading with lenses a lot, my eyes almost didn't react to them, and I wasn't succeeding in improving my focusing capacity.

I understood my mistake later on. I was reading the text wearing the lenses, but I was regulating the relationship of distance/lens dioptric power (+4.00 D in that time), allowing myself to read the text easily. What I was supposed to do was to increase the relationship of the lens dioptric power/reading distance and concentrate on focusing the induced defocus state, using CRB (Contraction/Relaxation/Blinking) movements. (See Chapter 5 for more on CRB.)

To gain improvements and to *accelerate* them, it's very important that the letters of the text we are reading while wearing training lenses are not in focus (in a retinal defocus state). Later on, the letters should be focused with CRB movements. The visual system reacts and gets used to the new refractive state by repeating focusing on each single word or letter, compensating for the initial functional refractive error. Each time we train our eyes with retinal defocus we should wonder, "At what distance will I be able to read today?" By doing so, retinal defocus progress, as well as the other adaptation and improvements, will be achieved.

Keep in mind: We are talking here about therapeutic defocus. That would be myopic defocus for myopia and hyperopic defocus for hyperopia. It is not a destructive or palliative defocus—which occurs when a myopic person views near with negative lenses and a hyperopic one with positive lenses. In such cases, an inauspicious accommodative stimulus—led by convergence—will find a further stimulus for increasing accommodative response.

Paradoxical Focusing: The Importance of Having Breaks between the Exercises of Defocus

The proximity of the observed object is one of the stimuli for the accommodative response. This occurs when we look at or view a near object. Two actions occur when we look closely:

1. The eye "accommodates" (adjusts the internal lens to reduce blur detected at the retina).

2. The eyes "converge" (adjust their position to reduce disparity between the images seen by both retinas).

For these reasons there is a close relationship among the observed object's distance, the visual axis's converging, and the accommodative response.

Under normal conditions, without optical modification due to external lenses, whenever the eyes converge the eye becomes myopic because of the cross-link relationship to the accommodation system. This is a normal physiological process and the only exception exists when a myopic person is training for myopic retinal defocus (with positive lenses) on the near text (within arm's distance). In this case (impossible in natural conditions, not faked with positive lenses for therapeutic purpose), the process of focusing, affected by the lenses and helped by CRB movements in the presence of myopic defocus, occurs in a *paradoxical* condition, together with eye converging.

In normal conditions, whenever converging, the eye becomes myopic, therefore causing accommodation to act—but when training with optically induced defocus (for therapeutic reasons and for acting over the accommodative balance), we are looking to decrease the accommodative response in the presence of convergence. It's much more useful to train with near-point retinal defocus (with suitable lenses) than with far-point retinal defocus. In the latter case, it would be necessary to run long distances (near or far from the observed object) so as to bring the eye to the state of slight retinal defocus.

So as to compensate for this condition of paradoxical focusing—paradoxical defocus that occurs in the presence of convergence—it is necessary to take some short breaks while working on focusing in the presence of optically induced retinal defocus. How to do such breaks? Relax your eyes by looking in the distance and do some eye rotations in both directions. By doing so, the stimulus for converging will be canceled, and your focusing capacity will respond to your training in retinal focus/defocus.

Chapter 4

Muscular Training
and Gradual Retinal Defocus

The focusing state of an emmetropic person (one with normal sight) is set up at "infinity"; that means that he or she can see clearly at medium and long distance and his or her eyes are not subjected to accommodative stimulus. This is the physiological state of the normal eye.

Accommodative stimulus—when focusing at near distance—occurs when the observed object comes nearer or is at a "near point." This is very important, since the mechanism of accommodation represents a stimulus for "pushing" the eye toward the myopic state. However, when resting, the eye focuses at infinity. That's why the process of accommodation is considered as active, and "disaccommodation" is seen as a passive process of relaxing your accommodation.

Accommodation is an active stimulus that leads to shifting from the physiological state of resting, where the accommodation is completely relaxed and focusing is at infinity. Prolonged near-work stress—accommodative stress—influences the eye's ability to get back to its physiological state of basic accommodative tone; that means resting.

Most myopia starts with excessive overaccommodative stress. Later, this stress becomes solidified because of wearing negative contact lenses. Shifting to the myopic state led by near-point stress can be observed easily, even in emmetropic people: it's enough to subject them to an efficient and prolonged accommodative stress, making them focus at a near object *for a long time*. Despite being different for each person, the result will be transient myopia. Ocular convergence increasing will worsen the overaccommodative state further (since convergence is a further stimulus for accommodation). In these cases, the right solution would be to relax the accommodation gradually and periodically, simply looking at far objects, or even better, at infinity.

Whenever it is possible, the overaccommodative stress should be limited, creating the state of light "blurring" with positive lenses or wearing undercorrection (for high myopia, where it is necessary to use negative lenses to view near).

Physiological Underaccommodation: The Wisdom of the Eyes

Accommodative stimulus reveals an inborn wisdom of our eyes and our body in general. Such mechanisms of physiological underaccommodation ("accommodative lag") result in an accommodative stimulus developed whenever we focus on something. This stimulus moves from a relaxed state (basic accommodative tonus) to clear the retinal image. This clearing action of accommodation allows us to see the most important details of the observed object.

Each time we focus on a near object, the accommodation that is going on in that very moment is lower than the one needed (considering the distance of the object). Therefore, there's always a "physiological underaccommodative" concerning the distance to the observed object.

This mechanism seems to be justified by the fact that our thrifty eyes use the accommodative stimulus wisely—to focus the observed object well—without arousing an excessive stimulus that could, with time, lead to accommodative overtone and, consequently, to myopia.

This "self-protective" stimulus is completely undermined by wearing minus contact lenses or glasses even at near distance. Wearing minus-lens glasses all the time will cause accommodative overtone. Myopes are advised to take off their minus-lens glasses when looking at near distance for this reason. The use of contact lenses is even worse because one cannot take them off whenever focusing at near distance—within the range where myopes normally can see well.

By knowing the SAID Principle, we can develop the advantages instead of disadvantages just by using it. As an alchemist once said, "So up as down." As refractive error could worsen, it could also be improved using the same principles but in an opposite way. How? Using positive lenses for myopes and negative lenses for hyperopes: in training sessions and normal life, but never when common sense and the law requires the use of full correction.

In this case, the load—accommodation, the natural system of focusing—will be stimulated and restored with time, with consequent natural regressing of the functional visual error.

The Way You Become Myopic

The use of corrective lenses solidifies and increases overaccommodative stress gradually. In times of hard mental and physical stress, after overaccommodative stress (for example, after studying for exams), you can notice some difficulties in focusing.

Rushing to an optician, you would be diagnosed as a low myope, which is always "corrected" by a "leisure" or a "part-time" minus lens. From this moment on, you become a "serious" myope, wearing those minus lenses, even being obliged to increase their strength every now and then, because of your ocular adaptation to the stronger and stronger minus lenses. This is a result of the SAID Principle (Specific Adaptation to the Imposed Demand).

All this is made worse by great ignorance about the rules of visual prevention: the simple rules of behavior that could prevent myopia from developing in the first place. For example, the kind of work being done—what is *extremely* harmful is reading at near distance wearing minus contact lens. This situation will produce *strong* overaccommodation. That is the reason why contact lenses bring about visual worsening. A myopic person who uses his glasses cleverly takes them off for reading and in near-distance activities—something impossible to do wearing contact lenses.

Minus Lens Glasses, Contact Lenses, and Refractive Surgery: Negative Use of the SAID Principle

In our "all and now" society, a patient who comes to an ophthalmologist wants to see well and *now,* without any effort. In my ten years of looking for perfect sight, I searched, over and over again, for a solution for my myopia. If someone had offered me a choice, an honest "fighting chance," it would have greatly shortened my struggle and efforts—and ultimately successful results.

According to the SAID Principle, every organ becomes accustomed to induced stimuli. A person who is using one substance constantly (for example, a drug) over time reacts to it less and less. The same thing happens in the case of physiological adaptation effected by external causes. The body becomes accustomed to lifting a load, generating muscular hypertrophy and neuromuscular adaptation in fiber recruitment.

The very same SAID Principle occurs in the case of wearing contact lenses (minus for myopes and plus for hyperopes). When wearing contact lenses a myopic person "freezes" his focusing system, making his eyes lazy and causing adaptation to the lenses *in pejus* (the negative one). It is also true that, after being diagnosed with myopia, people are given contact lenses until reaching full correction (10/tenths) with monocular vision, or even 11/tenths! It means that with binocular vision (without covering one eye) and at distances shorter than the ordinary prescribed for the ocular health examinations, *a person is in a state of overcorrection!*

With time, such a highly corrected state leads to *negative* adapting to that lens. After wearing a pair of new glasses with lens dioptric power equal to the last prescribed one, a person could be in trouble even looking at near objects like the floor, seeing it slightly deformed. When you ask an optician for an explanation, you are usually told, "Don't worry, you must get used to the new lenses." What a misleading statement. Your eyes "get used to that minus lens" by getting worse.

What does it mean? Being in a state of overcorrection, your eyes must even get used to the too-strong minus lenses that generate . . . *myopia!* This negative state of overaccommodation is worsened further with improper use of glasses: it develops when the myope (who is able to focus well at near distance) reads or works at near distance (near-work) wearing the glasses that would work well for viewing in distance. The result is the same: overcorrection leads to negative ocular adaptation and consequently generates myopia "spontaneously." Gradual worsening, which is usually noticed in myopes, could be prevented or slowed down if we would respect and following simple rules of visual hygiene as well as wearing positive lenses—before we begin wearing the minus lens.

Cure the Cause of Refractive Errors, Not Their Symptoms

Why is it that minus-lens glasses, contact lenses, and refractive surgery are not advisable for "curing" refractive errors? A solution for the problem could be transient, using a method that does not act on the *causes* of the problem itself. We can have a definitive solution. This solution involves intervening and eliminating the very same cause—namely, excessive close work.

The most evident example of a transient solution and treatment for myopia is wearing minus-lens glasses. These work instantly and convince most people that they must be the right answer. Casual use of this approach does not take into account that thoughtless use of such can worsen myopia. This occurs, specifically, when a myope reads and looks within the (near) range where he is normally able to focus *without* optical help—when you keep your minus lens on when reading. The minus-lens solution is transient since it does not act on the causes that generate myopia in the first place—the close work. The cause is weak ocular muscles produced by the close work and, consequently, the inability to focus on distant objects. The minus lens acts mechanically on refraction.

Refractive surgery acts the very same way as minus-lens glasses and contact lenses. That is, by mechanically generating a deformation and modification of the cornea. This is done to instantly produce focus on the retina. The point is this: at what price?

We can use the working of a camera as an analogy for human focusing—it's as if we wanted to *modify* the shape and bending of the objective lens so as to repair a broken focusing mechanism on an automatic focusing camera instead of working with it. The problem is that we can take off and change the camera's objective lens easily, but at the moment we *can't* do it with the human eye and its cornea and crystalline lens.

I would be pleased if I were able to instill the idea that before using drastic and, above all, irreversible minus-lens solutions, it would be better to try all the less invasive and cheaper solutions. Everlasting, excellent intellectual and physical sight for everyone!

How Can the Process Be Reversed?
How Can You Relax Accommodation?

One of the Power Vision System's fundamentals is to relax accommodation and decrease accommodative overtone. Such results can be obtained, inducing a slight myopic state, using positive lenses for reading—the phenomenon called "fogging." Such beneficial preventive work should be augmented with ocular stretching or working at the maximum range of the ocular muscles so as to restore correct convergence, fusing capacity, and correct focusing on the central fovea.

Flashes of Clear Vision

Continuing with your training and doing these exercises, at a certain point you will notice a sudden and completely unexpected flash of perfect vision. This is caused by the fact that your eyes, even temporarily, will start working correctly. These flashes of clear vision, at the beginning, will disappear easily, just by blinking. However, such flashes will stimulate you to continue the exercises, so that, little by little, increasing the strength and flexibility of your ocular muscles will produce "flashes" that last longer and longer, until you reaching the long-desired goal of clear sight and vision stabilization.

The improvements in focusing capacity are often sudden: it is as if the strength and flexibility of your vision increased at the same time as your muscular coordination reached a critical point and displayed themselves suddenly. You can notice this phenomenon more easily by choosing a very intense training program, because the quantity and intensity of the exercises bring about a more efficient training stimulus. And this stimulus then leads to adaptation and better focusing of your vision.

Clear Vision Stabilization—Joy and Frustration

The stabilization of a much clearer refractive state is to be reached gradually, when the flashes of clear vision become so frequent and long as to be your natural, real new sight. Going down this path you could perhaps be disappointed, since there's nothing worse than to achieve the desired result and then see it fading away. This is normal, however. Rome was not built in a day, and true vision restoration takes time and patience.

The flashes of clear vision will give you greater trust and enthusiasm, but it does take time to become stabilized. For this reason, you should check your own eyesight on the chart. Remember, 20/40 is legal for driving a car. If you exceed this level, you can continue to work toward 20/20. It does take persistence. If you vision "drops back," just get back into the routine of "pushing print" with a plus lens.

Those who choose the Power Vision System could notice no improvement in their visual functioning after two to three weeks of correct training and then suddenly *see* the benefits. During the periods of apparent "stalemate," in fact, our eyes are accumulating all the positive and beneficial stimuli that give positive results.

Until you notice the positive results of clear vision—better focusing until you experience flashes of extremely clear vision—it's very important to keep trusting the system and its physiological mechanisms and *persevere* in your exercising until the next step. It is also important that you imagine each "step" in your sight improvement. You are to be completely aware of this since you can see better, by day and by night. Imagine it as making a mosaic—you can't see the picture until you put in the last tile (which represents the "last straw"—the final stimulus that makes all the previous ones become visible). This last tile is the one that lets the training stimuli reach that "critical point."

You are trusting and groping in the darkness until reaching a "jolt" of improvement that you see for yourself. This is what is required to renew your motivation and enthusiasm: move toward one's own target of maintaining clear distance vision for life.

The Secret of Perfect Sight

The ciliary muscle, considered the lens responsible for the process of accommodation, is a smooth muscle, not subject to voluntary contractions; therefore it can't be trained voluntarily or consciously. On the other hand, there are extrinsic ocular muscles that are responsible for the process of focusing. Mental and physical stress and damaging habits (too much near-work) have as a consequence *in pejus* adaptation of these little muscles, with further sight worsening.

The same *in pejus* adaptation can be noticed in people: the musculature of those who do not exercise atrophies; a tennis player who strains only one hand gives a rise to a greater muscular imbalance between her right and left sides, created by the functional adaptation on the side she uses more.

The thoughtless use of minus-lens glasses can worsen already deteriorated sight. This initial slight nearsightedness is caused by habits like too much near-work compounded by reading at excessively close distances. Once prescribed and put on, even minus glasses for trivial myopia, such as –0.25 and –0.50 diopters, will lead to gradual vision worsening. The function makes the organ. The bespectacled student will be obliged "to make his own eyes walk with visual crutches" (his minus glasses) for the rest of his life.

It would be as if we wanted or were required to continue walking using crutches—even after some convalescence and we no longer needed them. How much motor functioning would we lose in walking? The choice is up to you.

Once we understand how the SAID Principle can stop the process of sight worsening, it is necessary to plan training that takes into account your specific needs. We turn to that in the next chapter.

Chapter 5

The Two Phases of Training

There are two phases of training that can help to improve your focusing gradually.

Phase 1

Exercises of *active static stretching* are to be carried out as often as possible during the day. They will condition your eyes to get used to working at a complete range of capable movement.

These exercises are intended to have a double training effect on your eyes, both as *active* training, generating strength increase of agonist muscles, and as *passive* training, causing a beneficent stretching of antagonistic muscles.

The Effects

After this visual training, the muscles will have greater mobility and consequently be better able to focus—since an emmetropic eye has to move over a myriad of points on the object to focus correctly. This is because the retina focuses on only one extremely limited point of the figure you want to see.

Such improvement in mobility and motor coordination is the result of greater muscular strength and flexibility. This is true in both the body and the eye. The lens is being contracted by flexible little muscles. These exercises improve this action and enable greater coordination and motor capacity—such as is needed to maintain very accurate vision.

Phase 2

You use your glasses in the opposite way to the one that causes your vision to get worse. The ordinary use of minus-lens glasses is to help clear distance vision by facilitating your eye's adaptation to the near environment. In the Power Vision System your plus glasses or an undercorrection are used to create an overload while training focusing muscles—with consequent adaptation and counterbalancing of the initial minus refractive status.

The Effects

Slightly overloading focusing muscles (slightly "pushing" the eye toward the "far" state by positive lenses) is a process of physiological adaptation to the training stimulus that is accomplished by your work. This method of pushing the eye to see distant objects must be carried out by using the CRB (Contraction/Relaxation/Blinking) system, described later in the chapter.

It is very important to understand that in the case of myopes, the accommodative mechanism is more or less atrophied. Therefore, it takes time to gradually restore the natural and physiological automatic focusing system to its former status.

Your first attempts in practicing the system of automatic accommodation (enhanced by CRB movements) may seem difficult. However, you must be sure that the focusing muscles will start working—at least a little—and with time these little movements will be enhanced until the moment your eyes become accustomed to this mechanism. At that point, in order to make progress, it is necessary to increase focusing distance gradually.

Technique

The Power Vision System develops positive adaptation of the accommodative system with consequent better vision. Improvement continues until you reach emmetropia—and that depends on your personal effort in carrying out the following techniques. It does take perseverance to do these exercises properly.

Active Static Stretching of the Oculomotor Muscles (Phase 1)

The myopic eye is characterized by a small motility and reduced dynamics relative to a normal healthy eye that has greater motility. This motility allows the eye to change to the points of the visual field very precisely and quickly.

The following stretching exercises bring about remarkable improvement in strength and flexibility in the coordination and convergence of the ocular muscles that are responsible for pointing at the objects of interest. They are called "active static," since any ocular muscle's stretching happens because of active and voluntary contraction of its agonist.

These exercises restore the perfect symmetry of agonist and antagonistic muscles that surround the eyes, thus keeping them in dynamic balance. This balance is required for precise and well-focused vision. Strained and contracted ocular muscles become more flexible and stronger through the execution of this kind of active static stretching exercise.

Improved muscular coordination has the advantage of bringing about better focusing, making the image fall onto the central fovea of the retina. The fovea is characterized by sharper focusing capacity in relation to the rest of the retina. This is where the entire image falls in case of weak coordination and convergence.

The Set of Ocular Stretching Exercises

The most important factor in these exercises is muscular work intensity. Gradual increasing of intensity leads to consistent training stimulus and physiological adaptation. This produces better coordination, resistance, and focusing after restoring natural shape to the normal ocular globe. The exercises are illustrated in Figure 5.1.

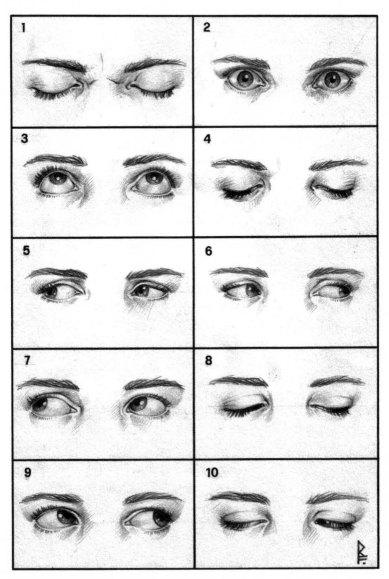

Figure 5.1   Ocular Stretching Exercises

1. Close your eyelids tightly *(without squinting your eyes)*.

2. Open your eyes wide (also your eyelids). *Keep in mind:* This exercise is also a part of the CRB movements.

3. Look up as far as you can.

4. Look down as far as you can.

5. Look to the right as much as you can.

6. Look to the left as much as you can.

7. Look up to the right decisively.

8. Look down to the left decisively.

9. Look up to the left decisively.

10. Look down to the right decisively.

Muscular work and constancy are the keys for improving your vision in doing these exercises.

Implementing These Methods

Stretching Variant for Rotations While Fixing at a Point

Fix at a point at more than 10 feet distance. Carry out head rotations, maintaining fixation and binocular fusion, until you reach the edges of your visual field. Binocular vision will tend eventually to double in some parts of visual field because of the strength and flexibility asymmetry of the agonist and antagonistic ocular muscles.

The goal is to carry out this rotation *at the edges* of the visual field while maintaining binocular vision. With time you will acquire it even in those parts where it was not possible before. This exercise leads to restoring not only the extrinsic ocular muscles' symmetry but also will bring about better convergence and fixation, which are necessary for precise and automatic focusing.

Important:

- Having ascertained which parts of visual field lack flexibility and strength, keep on doing the exercises. You should concentrate on the parts where more training is needed.

- Don't be afraid of forcing the rotation: the factor of muscular work intensity is the basic one for physiological adaptation of the oculomotor muscles and for the consequent increase in flexibility and strength. This is the fundamental factor needed to restore normal visual functioning.

Stretching Variant for Cyclorotations

The complete movement, made of the combination of 3, 7, 5, 10, 4, 8, 6, and 9, is the exercise of *cyclorotation.*

Carry out complete ocular rotations as if you wanted to follow the borders of a very big clock. Your head must stay still, without any rotation. You will notice a little resistance in some parts of visual field, due to low muscular flexibility and strength. Carry out these exercises until you feel the loosening of these "knots." With time and training you will achieve better ocular functioning.

The rotations must be carried out with closed and open eyes.

Important:

- Having ascertained which parts of visual field lack strength and flexibility, continue the exercises and determine the parts where more training work is needed.

- Don't be afraid to force rotation. Muscular work intensity is the basic one for physiological adaptation of oculomotor muscles and for their consequent strength and flexibility increase. These are fundamental factors for restoring the normal visual functioning.

- Your eyes could be stiff, most likely in the first days of doing the exercises with considerable force. Whatever the kind of intense work performed on a muscle, the effort generates a transient drop in its functioning that leads to adaptation to the training load, which in this case is generated by these rotations.

Training for Focusing

This kind of training has three variants, depending on the level of your myopia.

Variant 1

This variant is training without using corrective lenses (whenever you're able to make the letters slightly blurred by simply shifting the text to arm's length or bringing the text nearer to your eyes).

Variant 2

For myopes, this is training to focus by using positive lenses. For hyperopes, it's training to focusing by using negative lenses.

This variant is used for low myopia, whenever someone is able to read the text (a newspaper, for example) when holding it at arm's distance. In this case we must use stronger and stronger positive lenses to create slight "fogging" within a reasonable distance. In the case of hyperopes, we use the opposite procedure: we must use stronger and stronger negative lenses to create slight "fogging."

Variant 3

Training to focus by putting positive lenses *in front of* the usually worn ones. Placing positive lenses in front of negative ones, which are usually used for distance vision, is aimed at "downloading" dioptric power and stimulating the eyes to focus. People with high myopia, which doesn't allow them to carry out the first two variations, should practice with this one. The opposite works for farsighted people: put negative lenses in front of the positive ones. Undercorrected glasses can also be used.

How to Start?

For Myopia

1. Choose a printed text (a book, newspaper) and hold it in your hands as distant as necessary to have the letters in focus.

2. Shift the text until fogging occurs so as to make the letters hardly readable.

3. Then, open your eyes and eyebrows widely and decisively, for about 5 seconds (use CRB movements).

4. Relax your eyes; blink delicately.

5. Repeat the sequence throughout one training session.

Whenever carried out correctly, this procedure allows you to focus the text that was blurred at that distance previously.

Important: The text must be shifted little by little to create fogging, since without it the stimulus isn't enough to create positive adaptation. If you are not able to focus the text, perhaps it was shifted too much (the visual system perceives an excessive stimulus as something that is impossible to be focused).

In the beginning of training with this procedure you will hardly be able to focus the text and letters well because your oculomotor muscles are overcontracted and lacking in the strength and flexibility that let the focusing system work naturally and physiologically. The Power Vision System and its Basic Level Program (see Appendix 2) allows you to create the needed levels of strength, flexibility, and coordination.

This procedure is positive and provides useful training for the focusing system. Keep working with this exercise: open your eyes widely for about 5 seconds, with the text in front of your eyes, and relax them, blinking delicately.

For Hyperopia

1. Choose a printed text (a book or newspaper) and hold it in your hands as distant as necessary to have the letters in focus.

2. Bring the text nearer, very slowly, till slight fogging is created, where the letters are hardly readable.

3. Open your eyes and eyebrows widely and decisively, for about 5 seconds (CRB movement).

4. Relax your eyes; blink delicately.

5. Repeat the sequence throughout one training session.

This procedure, when carried out correctly, allows you to focus on the text that was blurred at that distance before.

Important: The text must be brought nearer gradually, so as to create fogging, since without it the stimulus isn't enough to create positive adaptation. If you aren't able to focus the text well, perhaps it was brought too near (the visual system perceives an excessive stimulus as impossible to be focused).

In the beginning of training with this procedure, you will hardly be able to focus the letters well. The oculomotor muscles are lacking in the strength and flexibility that allow the focusing system to work naturally and physiologically. The Power Vision System and its Basic Level Program (in Appendix 2) allows you to create the needed levels of strength, flexibility, and coordination.

This procedure is positive and constitutes useful training for the focusing system. Keep on doing this exercise over and over again: open your eyes widely for about 5 seconds with the text in front of your eyes, and then relax them, blinking delicately.

The CRB Movements (Phase 2)

The CRB movements, or Contraction/Relaxation/Blinking, is a system that encourages the eye to restore its normal accommodative capacity gradually. The eyes (eyebrows included) are to be opened widely and strongly and then relaxed in the focusing stimulus presence (wearing training glasses that create slight fogging, fixing on an object or signboard that is placed as distant as to be able to focus it after CRB movements).

The Physiological Explanation

A myopic eye is overloaded with chronic tension. In most cases, a myopic person doesn't recognize this tension since it is a part of his being and seeing. The fundamental factor for leading to muscular relaxation is to feel the tension and heighten it with another contraction. After that, let yourself go into local and general relaxation. Feeling a muscular contraction, then contracting the muscle strongly, and at the end relaxing it completely facilities relaxation both of the specific part and the whole body.

The CRB movements have their physiological basis in muscular relaxation induced voluntarily and consciously through preliminary contraction of the ocular muscle. In the case of myopia, the state of chronic contraction mostly strikes *musculus obliquus,* which keeps the eye in overcontraction and leads to progressive eyeball lengthening.

The eyeball lengthening is stressed further because of overaccommodation that creates hyperopic defocus and, in time, leads to physiological or structural adaptation and retinal shifting posteriorly. The condition of chronic muscular contraction is evident in many myopes whose glance looks "wide open" and less mobile. In this case the vision is not fluid and relaxed.

The CRB movements are aimed at facilitating relaxation (and, consequently, focusing during the exercises of myopic retinal defocus). Muscular contraction in CRB movements is carried out by opening the eyes wide and then relaxing them, annulling the contraction, to increase relaxation further with normal blinking. Natural and physiological eyelid blinking is more or less jeopardized in myopes by the state of chronic contraction that comes from wide-open and blocked eyes.

The value of the CRB movements is confirmed by Jacobson's Progressive Relaxation technique, which uses voluntary muscular contraction in different parts of body, followed with complete and prompt relaxation, so as to lead to the state of general relaxation. By feeling and increasing muscular contraction and then following it with prompt relaxation, you can change the state of muscular tension, causing muscular and general relaxation. CRB movement efficacy, together with suitable training for a specific kind of retinal defocus, must be preceded with preliminary preparation of ocular muscles through the exercises of active stretching and rotations at extreme parts of the visual field.

The Necessity of Accommodative Stimulus Presence

It's necessary to set up a stimulus together with CRB movements so as to achieve visual adaptation. Such necessity is based on the phenomenon of blur-driven accommodation.

A person, after training with the CRB system together with light stimulus for focusing, becomes used to having feedback for her capacity of focusing and is completely aware of being able to focus voluntarily where she wasn't able to do it previously. With time, a myope becomes used to "disaccommodating" (relaxing accommodation fully) and eliminating the overcontraction and overaccommodation that characterize his eyes, becoming able to focus ever further (till, eventually, he reaches the state of normal emmetropic sight).

Keep in mind: Such a real possibility of restoring clear, distinct sight is the goal of the Power Vision System. The duration of such a process depends on many factors, such as the degree of the initial myopia, training time (daily and weekly), training scrupulosity, one's emotional state, diet, and trust of the system (the real engine of the healing process).

The Bioenergetics' Explanation

According to bioenergetics, the human body is made of "nature's armor," one or more bodily segments characterized with conditions of muscular stiffness due to emotional and mental strains. The eyes are one of these parts, especially in people who suffer from visual errors. Such chronic muscular contraction leads to staring (in the case of chronic muscular contraction in the forehead and eyelids) and to changing the normal and physiological sphere shape of the eyeball.

According to Lowen (1994), fear—emotion coming from someone's childhood—is crystallized in such a block of one ocular segment: "An ocular segment releases from fear when someone, being frightened, opens his eyes wide and, then, his eyelids and forehead start moving again, showing off the emotions" (Lowen, 1983).

This movement is a CRB one.

Train Your Eyes and Then Forget Them

The process of accommodation as well as the process of vision are natural, instinctive, and unconscious processes. Training with lenses allows the experienced person to intervene over his process of accommodation voluntarily, despite the fact that it is ordinarily carried out automatically and with or without your intervention. The aim of the Power Vision System exercises—both muscular training (ocular rotations and fixing on a point at the edge of the visual field) and focusing—is to effect full ocular functioning as well as its complete rehabilitation.

After doing these exercises, it is important to allow your eyes to move freely without thinking of anything else but observing the object. Otherwise, the natural process of seeing would be hindered. In everyday life, focusing must be automatic and spontaneous, completely different from what happens in the exercises of focusing voluntarily with training lenses.

If it weren't so, we would risk both visual system overloading and perpetuating this state of tension instead of eliminating it. The rest and recovery after training sessions are as important as the training itself: too short a recovery time will not allow the optimal increase of muscular functioning and performance qualities.

After having trained our eyes well and suitably, we should "forget" them and let our eyes act freely and naturally, as they do instinctively. Having completely recovered after a training session, our sight will be strengthened and able to rely on the muscles that are strengthened as well.

Either Exercises or Habits? The Importance of Following the Correct Sequence

We often wonder whether visual training includes true exercises or simply the right visual habits. Many experts on visual rehabilitation state that some of these exercises shouldn't be considered only as "exercises," as something singular to be carried out only in visual training sessions, like relearning correct blinking, ocular shifting, or correct and full breathing.

A person must relearn these habits if he wants to increase his own visual capacities. Such habits must become a part of his "being" and eyesight. They are settled at the subconscious level of a person with normal sight—the very same habits that must be relearned by those who have refractive visual errors.

It is important to point out that these habits must enter the subconscious without any conscious personal effort—unless someone is repeating them voluntarily so as to make them become automatic. At the beginning, the habits like blinking, shifting, and deep and full breathing must be repeated mechanically—that's the way to feel them and be aware of doing them, since at that moment they aren't yet unconscious habits. Therefore, these exercises can't be considered as real and true ones, but as the correct ways of being and using one's eyes to be reestablished and carried out automatically and unconsciously all day long.

As to the exercises of muscular rehabilitation (like cyclorotations and fixing objects at extreme parts of the visual field), we can speak about true exercises. A person undergoing rehabilitation of a limb must move it at least until his limb musculature becomes as strong as to allow him full and physiological use of the rehabilitated limb. The movements of cyclorotation should be considered true and real exercises—the most important to bring about strength, flexibility, and restored muscular coordination in the visual system.

Without this kind of preliminary and basic work, even Bates's exercises (blinking, shifting) would be jeopardized. Full visual rehabilitation goes through different levels, and the first one is the work of restoring basic muscular qualities needed for doing more demanding tasks like blinking, shifting, or focusing with positive lenses.

Making exceptions or skipping the phase of pure and simple muscular work would be like, in the phase of rehabilitating an injured limb, trying to run before being able to walk. Let us provide an example from gymnastics. The exercises of high motor coordination, like double somersaults, at first begin with the basic muscular qualities (rising and leaping) trained gradually, and then, later on, specific exercises of rotation (at first on the springboard and then on the floor) are practiced.

That's the reason it's important to follow the correct sequence of the exercises and "habits" so as to gradually rehabilitate your natural sight. The Bates exercises, endowed with remarkable efficacy, produced even greater improvements in the people who were already working on improving their sight. This is possible if preceded by a period of pure muscular rehabilitation of the extrinsic ocular muscles, as described in the Power Vision System.

The very same thing will work with ocular biofeedback by use of the Accommotrac Vision Trainer, which provides sound feedback from a machine. This can have great benefits, because the treated person will have better control over her visual system by being able to better sense the variation in her focusing muscles.

Chapter 6

Stress

The Autonomic Nervous System and Sight

Getting the State of Comfort Back

The harmonious balance between the sympathetic and parasympathetic nervous system allows us to understand a great deal about the nature of the visual process—as a phenomenon related to someone's being and perceiving. Any imbalance between the sympathetic and parasympathetic nervous system can cause refractive problems. These are produced by a visual functioning deficit involving the level of tonic accommodation.

These factors must be used to evaluate the recovery time from near-work-induced refractive error. Intervening with respect to your refractive or focusing capacity at a near distance leads you to "normal vision" by gradually producing emmetropia. You could also intervene over your complete nervous balance, since the nervous system is the relevant issue that is responsible for your homeostatic level.

The homeostasis level reflects your capability of being in harmony with yourself and your environment. It is not by accident that an undesired refractive error highlights your psychophysical, behavioral, and relational differences. Such differences, obvious in the case of myopia or hyperopia, could be the result of a different balance or imbalance on the nervous level. The eyes are not only the windows of our soul, but also the filters through which we perceive our surrounding world. Our judgments and statements about our environment are created on the basis of these perceptions, and consequently, our actions are correspondingly adjusted.

Your perception of yourself and your surrounding environment is necessarily the sum of your thoughts and represents your world. Refractive capability is very important in such perceiving, since your sight is the first link to your surrounding world. You judge a great deal of your world on the basis of what you see. In fact you do this on your visual interpretation of what your eyes allow you to see, depending on their condition. If you are tired and have low energy, your eyes will suffer from it, and you will have a tendency to withdraw from the world. If you do not judge that you have a good visual experience with your environment, you cannot properly interact with the world in this circumstance. The right attitude toward solving difficult problems can bring about healing of the visual organs as a consequence. This occurs with issues that are beyond just the superficial "sight phenomenon."

The eyes are not like a car, but rather are part of a human being. If you wish to improve this fundamental system of perception, you must also improve your whole person. A person whose visual capacity has been improved becomes more able to "flow" in the life ocean. A person who is at peace with himself and with the entire world flows gracefully by his thoughts, actions, and interactions. This state of grace enables him to function at the highest level of creativity and being.

The level of being means the capacity of demonstrating your qualities, emotions, and your deepest personal desires. You can achieve this state when you understand your real priorities and your deepest needs. Your spirit must understand your own program of existence. Your "life script" makes you aware of your real needs as a person in development. It is when your spirit commits to a project, action, behavior, profession, or love that you are aligned with your own path. Only you can understand the quality of such experience. This attitude develops into a state of well-being—in health, creative harmony, and self-intelligence.

In the opposite case, whenever you feel that an undertaken experience or action isn't beneficial, then you "put your foot down" and resist advocacy for change. Physical symptoms and apparently accidental circumstances are the signs that will take you back to the "right way." The right way is always the way of our heart—whether we are aware of it or not.

The heart is the barometer of our feelings and our deepest emotions. When our heart beats strongly because of an emotion, it wants to tell us something. The person who acts in a manner that (to him) has a "heart," the person who listens to her heart signals, full of emotions, is on the right way to reach the state of "grace of being."

The eyes, as the windows of our soul, show off this state of grace and our level of connection with ourselves. The eyes can also shine with true and real emotions. Even physically, the eyes are the point that is in the most direct touch with the brain (by optic chiasma, which is a part of the brain system).

Working on rebalancing our eyes consequently leads to the autonomous nervous system (sympathetic and parasympathetic) rebalancing. Our homeostatic level as well as our inner equilibrium and the possibility of our being in a "high-quality" state depends on this fact. The opposite is true as well: working on the nervous system brings about better vision of ourselves and the entire world.

This is the point where the visual reeducation system starts, aimed not only at physical sight strengthening but also at strengthening one's inner and outer perceptions.

Mental Stress and Ocular Relaxation

Perfect sight can be achieved only through relaxation.
—W. H. Bates

The great pioneer in objecting to the use of minus lens was Dr. W. H. Bates, who established a healing method based on his judgment of mental relaxation. Once achieved, mental relaxation reflects on all bodily functions, including the extrinsic ocular muscles. Therefore, one's general relaxation (including the eyes) is the necessary condition for optimizing one's focusing ability.

Such a relationship between mental and ocular tension—as Bates stated—is backed up by modern theories on myopia development (see Skeffington, 1974/1928; Birnbaum, 1985, 1993). According to this theory, our modern society, requiring much near-work, leads people to many different refractive errors (particularly myopia).

Skeffington postulated that long periods of intense concentration, immobilization, and mental effort, associated with near-work (like studying, reading, and other cognitive processes) lead to the focusing system adapting to very short distances—with the eye developing a negative focal status as a consequence. Birnbaum (1984) admits to the value of Skeffington's theory on "proximal stress" and explains the visual system's adaptation to a confined environment by activating neuro-endocrine mechanisms that are associated with stress (see Cannon, 1929).

This type of stress mechanism is activated by increased activity of the sympathetic nervous system, which normally acts on the basis of "fight or flight." Many scholars have supported the close relationship between stress (induced by sympathetic nervous system stimulation) and the effort that accompanies visual attention (see Kahnemann, 1973; Libby et al., 1973; Pribram & McGuinness, 1975).

This type of stress occurs during high cognitive processes as described in Hess and Polt, 1964; and Beatty and Wagoner, 1978. The basis of the near-point stress theory is the negative adaptation of refractive system to ever-closer and stressing engagement—that is, that modern people engage in many near-distant activities. These long hours of near-work do not "work" with normal physiology that requires well-balanced visual situations, such as distance work as opposed to hard and stressful near-work.

This creates a situation of general stress in people and, with time, produces a negative focal adaptation with the most widespread consequence—myopia. The proximal stress theory must be included together with other physical stimuli—that is, the eye must be treated as a "system." Therefore the eye's focal status must be considered in concert with physiological and mental stress. The visual system is subjected to stress such as overconvergence and overaccommodation. In Bates's theory, myopia is a result of mental stress and could be largely ended by recognizing these basic concepts. The concept that the eye is behaving as a "system" is strongly supported by recent studies.

Relation between Mental and Ocular Muscles' Tension

As Bates postulated, a part of our focusing and adjustment ability is determined by the six external ocular muscles. Their overcontracting leads the ocular globe into a situation of permanent deformation. This deformation, then, leads to an error in focusing an image on the retina.

This thesis is correct as determined by studies conducted by more recent scholars. Some suggest that the ocular globe axis lengthens and therefore must produce a focusing error, that is, myopia. This is the result of a chronic isometric contraction of the extrinsic ocular muscles as a part of the general ocular tension caused by attention and problem solving. The problems that are ascribed to using or abusing mental and cognitive processes are the real reason the eye adapts its focal state to a "near" environment by "going negative."

In brief, a myopic person is a person who is too stressed and too concentrated on his mental processes to relax and clear his distance vision by that process.

The Opposite Approach to Muscular Relaxation: The Key for an Efficacious Ocular Musculature Relaxation

Although Dr. Bates's thesis is correct, many people (including me) have made very slow progress in achieving muscular relaxation of the extrinsic muscles. This consequently led to slow improvements in focusing ability and reduction of my own myopia. We need to understand how to induce relaxation of the striated bodily muscles so we can explain with one precise reason why clearing distance vision is a slow process.

There is a close relationship between muscular strength and its capacity of lengthening, and therefore, relaxing. When a muscle is strong and well trained, it is able to demonstrate great flexibility and relaxation.

More or less atrophied muscles (myopes have such kinds of muscles) tend to have slower saccadic ocular movements, and this tends to deform the ocular globe axially. As opposed to this situation, strong and elastic muscles are able to work efficiently from a dynamic perspective (increasing and optimizing the saccadic movement and capability of pointing the objects) and from a static point of view (without deforming the ocular globe axially).

Relaxation through Muscular Work

One of the secrets for getting a muscle to relax is to increase its capability of active working throughout an ever-greater working range. A mistake is to insist on relaxing a nearly atrophied muscle with little strength and flexibility; it would hinder progress and slow down muscular working improvements and consequently would interfere with whatever focusing ability remains.

Muscular atrophy cannot be treated with relaxation but through muscular rehabilitation. This requires specific work that involves muscular fibers that work while they are contracting and extending.

Trying to relax the eyes with ordinary muscular relaxation procedures leads to limited benefits—since these procedures do not substantially act on muscular qualities like strength and lengthening. The only result is that we get a little reduction of chronic contraction.

How do we train our ocular muscles efficiently to rehabilitate them to a state of dynamic relaxation? What could we do and how could we gradually decrease the grip of overcontracted ocular muscles? How do we allow a gradual decreasing of axial lengthening, which caused the blur in the first place? How could we decrease chronic eye contraction and resultant wide-open myopic eyes? How could we restore the fluid ability of saccadic movements and central fixation? These targets can be reached through active muscular work at ever-higher ranges within the visual field. These are the exercises of ocular rotation: cyclorotation (described in Chapter 5).

No rehabilitation therapist would ever think of healing a chronically immobilized and atrophied muscle (for example, a muscle in a cast) by "relaxing" it. This work must be aimed at rehabilitating the muscular qualities like strength, flexibility, and coordination. As for the oculomotor muscles—which are chronically contracted within limited working range (as imposed by glasses)—our task must be to restore their muscular properties by working at maximum range (where focusing should happen). This must occur within all the visual field and not only in that little part that is limited by the frames of glasses.

This is the reason that active static stretching exercises (as described in Chapter 5) are used for training extrinsic ocular muscles in the Power Vision System. These exercises are to be carried out symmetrically and within *all* the ranges of ocular movement. Such work will allow the eyes to keep the glance relaxed (since the muscular qualities allow the muscle to work easily) and, at the same time, to optimize focusing by optimizing central fixation and saccadic vibration movements.

The Emotional Component in Myopia

Myopia is direct result of an emotional imbalance. This is true except in some very rare cases of congenital disorders of the visual organs at the structural level. Slight nearsightedness is a functional adaptation *in pejus*—in the case of near-work. Despite the fact that few myopic people are willing to admit it, in many cases, a myopic person can't see because—at least at an unconscious level—he doesn't want to see.

The reasons for such choice (however unconscious) are as many as the natures, situations, or personal experiences that you may have. The body and its organic functioning are shaped by what the mind thinks of itself at a subconscious level. Literally, and reasonably, we can state that someone can do only what he believes he can, as well as the opposite—the limited ideas are materialized, being literally bodily somatized as a psychosomatic disease.

Let us determine what the myopic person does not want to

see in his surrounding environment—and what, subconsciously, causes him to give up focusing naturally and correctly on distant objects. Psychotherapist Alexander Lowen, in his work *Bioenergetics* (1994) states that a possible explanation could be that the person is not willing to meet someone's glance—which could belong to either an authoritarian mother or a strict teacher. Another possible explanation for myopia development is the emotional pressure in bearing someone's glance. It is the case of a shy person. In many cases, such a person tends to develop an introspective and more or less isolated character—the so-called myopic character.

A strong emotion, repeated over time, creates muscular tension, which could be somatized in local muscular blocks. In myopia, such a block happens at the level of the ocular muscles, jeopardizing their correct and fluid functioning. It is as though we wanted to play piano with chronically contracted hands and fingers. Since the visual process is the result of perfect ocular muscles' synergy, it's easy to understand that clear, distinct vision is jeopardized by any tension at the ocular level.

It's important to speak about the emotional component in myopia since it lets us understand that either reducing or resolving such a component leads to positive change from psychological and behavioral points of view. Little by little you will be able to see "over" your former focusing distance. You will notice also that your former myopic vision of life is being dissolved.

You will further notice that you are more willing to deal with people and focus on their personalities. The quality of all your social contacts will improve. The eyes are the organs that put us in touch with our environment and people, more than any other organ. It is important that we improve their functioning and efficiency so that we can achieve better personal, emotional, and social results. The eyes are not only perceptive but also interactive organs.

Myopia, Power Vision, and the Strength of Glance

There's a huge difference between a glance "lost in the distance" that doesn't fix on anything and one that is concentrated "looking" at something—an object, a point, or another glance. Any myope has his own limit beyond which everything is blurred (or he doesn't see at all). Over that limit, the gaze is directed somewhere but doesn't fix. Therefore, myopes have an "undecided and powerless" glance, since they, literally, don't know what to fix on nor look at.

Myopia is often associated with an imbalance concerning muscular strength and flexibility. One ascertained, asymmetry (or imbalance) will determine both "central fixation" (therefore also focusing) and your ability to fix on any point surely and strongly. After being trained in static strength position and at extreme points of the visual field, the ocular muscles will develop better ability in "symmetric converging"—or fixation. All that will lead to better vision and a strong, sure, and concentrated glance.

A person's strength could be determined from their musculature. Bodily muscles are the "exposed" ones, and therefore visible. Your strength can be judged by a simple glance. So, how do the ocular muscles (the striated type, like the triceps muscle) express their strength if they are hidden and invisible, around the globe of the eye?

The answer is double: by focusing as well as fixing ability and by concentrating the gaze on a point. Such abilities can be remarkably improved through the ocular muscles' training according to the guidelines of the Power Vision System.

The secret for having a strong and powerful glance is in training the eyes and fixing during conditions of loading. You concentrate your glance to fix on a point (for example, in the middle of your eyes) at maximum ocular range (rotating your head symmetrically and circularly, thus keeping on fixing at a point). By doing these exercises, your ability to concentrate your glance increases, and ocular asymmetries disappear.

Chapter 7

Breathing

Its Importance and Therapeutic Potentiality

The breathing process (considered as one of the most ordinary and automatic bodily functions) hides one of the greatest mysteries of humanity: physical, mental, emotional, and therapeutic potentialities. Many great works on this issue have been written by oriental religions' "enlightened ones" and great scholars of occidental science.

What is important now is to understand the breathing phenomenon in relation to the functioning of our visual organs as well as to our ability of seeing. All this goes beyond the physical health of an organ itself and touches your "willingness to see" from an emotional point of view as well as from possible somatizations due to repressed and never-shown feelings such as fear, anxiety, and so forth.

As bioenergetics teaches us, the eyes have always been considered to be the soul's windows, and they are the most sensible means to demonstrate our feelings and our emotional state. Whatever passes through our eyes goes further than the light rays or the images.

The emotional richness of an image creates in its receiver a perception that goes beyond perceiving color, space, or the shape of the object. The emotional power of some images or some feelings can literally, over time, change someone's level of visual perceiving: think of "wide open eyes," the expression of a child's fear at seeing his mother's or his teacher's austere glance. Over time, such a position will cause a stillness and ocular bulb deformation, which leads to myopia. The physiological or mechanical result is a subconscious "unwillingness to see" and excluding the images from one's perception.

If this statement works well for visual functioning, then try to imagine all the subliminal devastation that most people are subjected to every day. Over time, such devastation turns into the most despairing pathologies.

Breathing, Psychosomatic Equilibrium, and the Eyes

How does breathing affect our eyes? Any emotion influences the nervous system, causing physiological alterations like blood pressure increasing, heartbeat varying, pupils contracting and dilating, breathing frequency and intensity changing. Homeostasis and psychosomatic equilibrium undergo great modifications: despite our body's natural tendency to restore its equilibrium when the stimulus is over, the nervous system's excessive stimulating may lead to the state of chronic "alert" and consequently to chronic psychosomatic stress. Correct and full breathing is the most natural and probably the most efficient antidote to take our body, mind, and soul back to the state of natural equilibrium.

Almost all people are wrong in thinking that they breathe correctly, "as they have always done," but they are not aware of being in a cage, made of a rigid bodily armor, that is the result of previous unobserved psychosomatic reactions and all the emotions and feelings imprisoned deep down at the bottom of their consciousness. That's the reason why, when someone starts breathing fully with his lungs and "being" he is "born again."

Many occidental schools on breathing take their name from such processes as Rebirthing and Vivation.

Learning fluid and natural breathing (free from blocks and inhibitions) is a cathartic and delicate process that leads to positive and deep changes in one's being. Such an ability is so great that we can compare it to learning to play an instrument (piano, for example); the highest goal is the supreme mastery in "playing" one's own breathing on a wave of deep personal inspiration (literally, inspiring inside).

I advise you to study and constantly use this "breathing issue," studying either from specific books or directly, from your own experience with professional teachers of Rebirthing, Vivation, and Pranayama yoga.

Circular Respiration

Among many yoga breathing techniques, I advise you to learn and use "circular breathing," as rebirthing and vivation suggest. Your breathing must flow in continual sequence, circulating without interruptions. Only practice, constant use, and trust will bring out the extraordinary potential of breathing power as well as of development, preservation, and vital energy use.

Keep Your Body in Homeostasis

When the body is in equilibrium, it is also in "homeostasis," where all the systems, especially the nervous system, work very efficiently. Whichever kind of interference acts on various bodily systems in this state of psycho-physiological equilibrium (cardiovascular, neurovegetal, endocrine system), it causes more or less evident bodily responses. Any kind of long-lasting stimulus leads either to adapting or to negative overloading. Everyone has his own threshold over which an excessive stimulus (whenever the body considers it so) produces a breach in the state of physiological equilibrium (homeostasis).

The eyes are the organs most affected by such imbalance and show it through function disorders. Such a statement has a dual physiological foundation: the first one is in the fact that the ciliary muscle is a smooth type and therefore is not subjected to voluntary contractions. The smooth muscles are influenced by the nervous system. Any type of alteration producing an excessive nervous stimulation also causes stress: many times such stress becomes a psychosomatic reaction or somatization of the ciliary muscle. It means that the muscle is not able to relax nor to focus the images correctly on the retina. In such a state, the ciliary muscle develops a spastic contraction, thereby creating a state of perpetual accommodation. This is one of the causes of myopia. Therefore, any condition that either reduces or eliminates the state of nervous and physiological overload is beneficial for vision.

The second physiological foundation is seen in the fact that some stimuli (which are stressing the nervous system) have repercussions on the state of chronic contraction of the bodily musculature (the striated muscles) and especially on the muscles around the ocular globe. Such an overtone, induced by repeated stress, with time leads to the ocular globe deforming and inevitably produces a focusing error.

How does one maintain homeostasis? The main indications to take into account are the following:

1. Maintain a balanced diet, avoiding as much as possible, food that produces a metabolic rate increase, like simple carbohydrates with a high glycemic index (that is, pure sugar, sweets).

2. Avoid stimulants like tea and coffee as much as you can.

3. Limit the quantity of alcoholic beverages.

4. Help your body and mind remain free from stress over-loading; practice simple relaxation techniques and mental clearing. This will include respiration (Rebirthing, Vivation, Pranayama yoga), physical exercises (especially aerobics), pro-gressive relaxation (Jacobson), autogenous training (Schultz), and meditation (see Holt, Caruso, & Riley, 1978).

There are an endless number of techniques, and usually whatever has a positive impact on the nervous system is also useful: even the *idea* of walking in the woods and along the seashore has a rebalancing power.

Expand Your Vision, Strengthen Your Sight

You must strengthen your insight—all that you believe as possi-ble or impossible in your world—so as to strengthen your vision. Your world and your horizons are the mirror of what you con-sciously or unconsciously believe is possible—personal relations, professional success, health, and wealth.

Our sight isn't different from this at all; it is the perception of our inner limits. If you are reading this book, accepting the possi-bility of innovative ideas on self-healing and clearing your sight, you are already encouraging yourself to overcome the limits that today's society has imposed on you.

Each and every day you crash into the "myopic mindset" and the widespread opinion that little or nothing can be done to pre-vent nearsightedness. Even a few academic authorities support this opinion. The widespread and accepted opinion on the use of "glass prostheses" (glasses) cannot be defeated—even when direct experimental data argues against it. The glasses are regarded as a sign of modern style. Again, the goal of the optical industry is to have you believe that there is nothing else you can do except wear minus-lens glasses.

If you reject this common idea and feel that there must be something better you can do for your eyes and for your level of perception, then you have already moved toward a correct and more effective method. Your wish and your idea of clearing your vision has led you to this book—and others—that are aimed at giving you the understanding and your eyes the natural power they originally had. Your goal is indeed to free yourself from negative-lens palliatives and therapeutic posturing. The objection is that these palliatives, though working "instantly," only make matters worse in the long run—and you have every right to know about the proven effect of the negative lens on the refractive status of the eye.

Most likely you are already learning and practicing the techniques established as part of the Power Vision System. You are increasing your focusing ability, and you can feel how your inner horizons are being opened up and your behavior is changing.

The eye's control process is bidirectional. The synergistic working on your eyes and strengthening their focusing ability provides the positive feedback that is so important for your visual future. When you see your distance vision clearing—by checking your own eye chart—you will be encouraged to continue with your efforts.

Therefore, your initial willingness is needed to clear your incipient myopic vision. Each human conquest (from scientific to spiritual knowledge—beyond the limits of common perception) has always been carried out by pioneers who overcame the limits imposed by social beliefs. They were courageous enough to go beyond (at the price of overturning the certainties and dogmas of those who accepted limited worldviews).

The Power Vision System allows you not only to see a beautiful landscape and a friend's greeting—but also to extend the limits of your being. These limits could be removed once you strengthen and heal your sight, after passing through the ocean of prejudices that are inhibiting you from taking such a step and achieving such a result.

What kind of spirit must you have to face your new task, being aware that any limit could exist if you accept it? What are the real limits of human progress? My friend, the answer is up to you. You will have the pleasure of overcoming your own limits, climbing onto a new life and perceptive horizons. Keep on trusting in improvement, as if it were a law of the world you are living in.

Healing Tears: The Curative Power of Crying

The eyes are the organs of visual perception and interaction, and their importance surpasses simple vision. The glance is our favorite channel through which we interact with the world. Our capability of flowing and living with others depends a great deal on our eyes. The mouth can lie, but not the eyes: the more pure the eyes are, the more able they are to express your deep feelings and emotions—which can't be expressed with words.

We can understand the great importance of clear and distinct vision when we completely understand the importance of emotions—which not only can create but also can destroy, with all the consequences on the psychological and physiological states. That's why we should keep these sensory organs (the eyes) in their pure primordial expression. The eyes of an open person (who is able to get his own emotions to flow freely) are calm and relaxed, as if they were the water's surface, able to reflect the images. Such a quality can be noticed within children, who are free from social conventions and expectations about being accepted, demonstrating their entirely innocent transparency.

Growing up, a child becomes a part of society in which feelings are less important, and indeed, every society gives less importance to expressing feelings and their power and cares more about repeating rules and social conventions. A social human being, loaded with conventions, duties, and targets for high social position and wealth, forgets about his inner reality—what would make him improve from a human point of view. Very often, a human being forgets that he is a person who is evolving. It happens when he lives his life and is doing his best to fulfill all the conventions and expectations imposed him by our society.

Very often we live someone's else life, putting aside our own needs to grow and evolve. Such a split between our needs as social beings and our personal, true needs creates cracks in our social, psychological, and physical well-being. Such a state could be demonstrated at a superficial level (a state of light dissatisfaction that is growing behind a comfortable and an apparently successful life) or more clearly as a state of organic weakening that could become an actual disease. Some people think that the eyes are the weakest ring in a chain of splitting between the social and superior Ego. Such people are the first to lose touch with their lives and get into blur, which testifies to their subconscious wish to detach from reality. This detachment makes the eyes hard and unable to express themselves and to interact completely.

Such eyes are unable to show off all their emotions, hidden under a hard expression—unable to communicate through their natural transparency. In this state of unconscious closure toward the world, together with deep personal expectations and desires imposed by a superior Ego, a person finds herself imprisoned and isolated in a visual fog that separates and oppresses her. At this point, unable to interact fully (from a perceptive and emotional point of view), the eyes gradually harden and somatize this state of disjointedness from the deep self and the surrounding world.

At this point, a person becomes unable either to cry or to get in touch with his surrounding world through his small, still part that perceives and sees everything but is now stifled by a distressed personality, formed by social expectations and conventions. Crying can make a person reborn toward a new insight and outsight: each tear (once hidden and held back) would open a new life toward seeing and embracing the world with grace and interacting with other people.

Crying is like knocking down the walls of a dam in front of a rushing river of feelings, which (when expressed) lead a person to integration, joy, and comfort never felt before. Soft eyes and a fluid glance are the result of inner transparency that reflects as visual ability, which can't work without real and authentic feelings, desires, and expectations of that still part (which is beyond the eyes themselves) desperately looking to be recognized. Crying is one of the best means of visual healing because it acts directly on the feelings of separation that have caused blurred sight.

Chapter 8

Other Methods

The Bates Method

No text on visual reeducation can avoid dealing with the work carried out in the early twentieth century by an ophthalmologist from New York, Dr. William Horatio Bates. He devoted a great deal of his life to developing natural methods of treating visual disorders through appropriate exercises and relaxation. He stated that standard treatments, like the use of a minus lens for "correcting" refractive errors, were completely wrong. He stated that ocular muscular stress and tension were the main reasons for the development of these errors.

Does Dr. Bates's Method Work?

Bates's method and its exercises established the basis for visual reeducation, but, speaking from my personal experience, the method gives much better and faster results if combined with the Power Vision System. Such a statement is based on the fact that the Bates Method points out the importance of relaxing oculomotor muscles but not the necessity of training them.

Physiological and functional properties of weak muscles that are more or less atrophied have low flexibility and strength as well as low resistance to stress. Dr. Bates's exercises (palming, swinging, and so forth) tend mostly to relieve the ocular muscles' chronic tension without acting directly to restore the physiological properties

107

(like strength, flexibility, resistance, and muscular coordination) that characterize a healthy eye. Though Bates's exercises bring about sight improvement, they don't grant substantial improvements like more intense exercises: for example, fixation, peripheral fusion, CRB (Contraction/Relaxation/Blinking) movements, using training lenses, and static active stretching exercises.

As any physician or sports trainer knows, the physiological factor of intensity in muscular training is the one that creates an effective stimulus for the trained muscles' adapting and consequently for the functional adaptation of the organ that is subjected to the stimulus. Bates's method is a limited one, and its limiting factor is the training stimulus intensity and, consequently, the results.

Undoubtedly, combining Bates's exercises with muscular training and progressive retinal defocus, we can have a more complete and efficient program for visual rehabilitation.

Biofeedback: Accommotrac Vision Trainer

The biofeedback technique is based upon the fact that many physiological functions that are ruled by the nervous system (for example, pupil opening and the process of accommodation) use a kind of servomechanism to adjust their response to a changeable condition. This system has been used worldwide to allow the treated person (with the help of a particular machine) to get control over certain organic functions that are often considered involuntary.

A group of researchers (Trachtman, 1978, 1981, 1986) proposed a technique aimed at letting the treated person get control over the process of accommodation. The system is called Accommotrac Vision Trainer and is made up of a box, display, and some buttons. A person who has difficulties in accommodating and focusing reeducates his ocular system by using the machine, which is equipped with a "test/error/visual-sound feedback" system. Such training is aimed at controlling the focusing system voluntarily, with consequent better visual functioning.

Does the Accommotrac Work?

The system works well and is based upon science about biofeedback. From my own twenty-sessions-long experience, I can confirm that at the end of each session I had positive results, but, unfortunately, my improvements were gone very soon after finishing the session.

A Supposition

The reason why my improvements were transient comes from the fact that the Accommotrac accustoms you to "disaccommodate" your myopic focusing (to relax the accommodation), bringing about relaxation of the ciliary muscle, which is overcontracted due to excessive overaccommodative stress (the main reason for functional myopia), but it does not directly act on restoring the physiological eyeball to sphericity (the eyeball is deformed by contracted and strained extrinsic ocular muscles).

To restore the extrinsic ocular muscles' function, we must train the muscles directly and restore (through suitable exercises) their flexibility, strength, and coordination. Training with a machine, you must maintain your glance fixed in a central position; this is opposite to the principles of ocular training at maximum range of movement, as described in the Power Vision System (PVS).

The results one usually achieves in training with Accommotrac would surely be much better if this visual rehabilitation technique were associated with exercises of muscular rehabilitation, as described in the Power Vision System. Stronger and more flexible muscles are more able to work dynamically and precisely.

Any kind of visual reeducation is aimed at rehabilitating the visual organ that suffers from functional disorders as well as at restoring specific properties of a healthy eye. The key words in visual reeducation systems are *training* and *adaptation*. A desperately needed basic is a direct and specific stimulus to create physiological adaptation. Such a stimulus acts on the organ (the eyes), aiming at creating the functional modification.

Training with the Bates Method is aimed at relaxing the nervous system and at rehabilitating the extrinsic muscles through specific exercises. Biofeedback is aimed at reeducating the system of accommodation, getting the person to be aware of his own capability of intervening in visual process. The Power Vision System acts through specific stimuli and loads.

- The load (the specific stimulus that allows the organ to create an adaptation) is the fundamental factor for success in training with all these systems. It means visual acuity stimulation.

- There's no adaptation without a specific stimulus.

Pinhole Glasses or Glasses with a Stenopaeic Hole

This kind of glasses, with many little holes and without lenses, uses the principle of the Stenopaeic hole, which "cuts" peripheral rays of light, making only their central part fall onto the retina and bring about better focusing.

Improvement depends on the eye viewing through one single Stenopaeic hole; in this case it means through just one among many Stenopaeic holes on the glasses. Therefore, the improvement is transient and completely depends on wearing glasses. After taking them off, since your focusing system hasn't been subjected to stimulation that may justify any lasting change in focusing, any improvement soon disappears.

There's no adaptation without a specific stimulus.

Which kind of adaptation do such glasses produce with time? Or, are the eyes able to see better taking off these glasses, since visual acuity has been stimulated (as it happens with suitable lens-driven retinal defocus)? Maybe the eyes or extrinsic muscles are stimulated by a kind of ocular "gymnastic" because the eyes must search for the holes to view, therefore increasing ocular mobility?

The improvement we've been discussing—the ocular muscles' functioning is restored by working at maximum range of ocular movement—doesn't happen (nor could it) through wearing glasses, including the pinholes ones.

About pinhole glasses, Rasterbrille, or the glasses with Stenopaeic holes, we point out the following:

- Such glasses don't create any adaptation to correct focusing; therefore they don't stimulate any kind of adaptation that could last after taking them off.

- Pinholes glasses don't create muscular adaptation that would improve visual functioning, since they imprison the glance and ocular mobility as much as any other kind of glasses.

I don't believe in the possibility of healing refractive errors with these glasses, since they are a kind of "addiction" that is completely strange to the eyes. Whatever creates any dependence can't be called curative.

The use of training lenses with PVS is justified by the fact that such lenses are aimed at acting beneficially on the refractive state through the principle of progressive retinal defocus and, eventually, at eliminating the refractive error completely.

My advice to people who would like to improve their focusing: Avoid all easy solutions and interventions; take on the responsibility for intervening over your refractive error through visual training, which requires long-lasting motivation.

We humans have already been given plenty of whatever we need for living on Earth. Glasses aren't needed—least of all the Stenopaeic ones.

Chapter 9

The New Age of Visual Reeducation

Everyone is the best doctor for himself.
—Hippocrates

Natural healing of refractive errors occurs through education and informing people of their personal responsibility for their own health. More importance should be given to prevention rather than treatment.

Yet, any disease is viewed as something that happens beyond your will, despite preventive medicine and simple rules of living (correct diet, physical training, suitable vitamins, stress lessening) that could bring about not only the decrease of psychosomatic disease (like refractive errors) but also increasing the level of personal well-being and living standards. Thus, health does not mean absence of disease, but a state of complete well-being concerning all personal aspects (emotional, mental, bodily). Such health conditions would lead to a higher levels of well-being and "being," including more creativity and more easily dealing with your environment.

All the benefits of a holistic treatment go far beyond symptom relief. After eliminating the causes of imbalance and having rehabilitated the organ or physiological system and returning to the initial level of efficiency (visual training in this case), a person feels as if he were reborn—with a new awareness and perception of himself and the entire world. In this case, "knowledge is power"—the power of influencing your own health and well-being by your lifestyle.

Each of us should be aware that it is up to us to motivate ourselves to develop healthy lifestyles, and that neither a pill nor a pair of glasses is enough to protect a person from disease. A new medicine, which isn't based only on healing symptoms but foresees a global healing of the entire person and informs her of her ability to be responsible for her own health, will lead to a new society: not only a more healthy society from a bodily point of view but also a more creative, healthy, and sane society from any point of view.

Functional Refractive Errors: The Review of Treatments

For how long have the traditional branches of medicine been ignoring the obvious causes of myopia? These branches are still supposed to treat myopia, which is reaching epidemic proportions—indeed becoming a social disaster. For how long will we be prescribed contact lenses without them making a difference, nor our doctors informing us about intervening by ourselves?

For how long will we, our children, and our grandchildren be victims of ignorance on this issue? Modern society could have correct statements on refractive errors if politicians or leaders in health care intervened. Maybe, such revolution in the optic industry could be born, informing and awakening every single person who is interested in really treating his or her own sight.

The project of informing people of their power and the possibilities of preventing or, at least, decreasing the spread of myopia, should contain the following phases:

- Informative campaigns by competent health bodies (commercials, magazines, special TV broadcasts)

- Distribution of brochures with necessary information

- Financing of scientific works on the natural treatment of refractive errors, including the works aimed at establishing standard procedures for each level of refractive error (large samples are lacking now; so it's impossible to set up and precisely standardize all the parameters for treating each group of people or level of vision defect)

- Establishing specialized centers (for preventive work and treatment)

- Encouraging prescription and the use of positive (plus) lenses for myopes, subsidizing the patients for free

Deceptive Advertising by the Vision Business

Sometimes you see on TV or in banner headlines, glossy magazines, or advertisements: "March—Sight Preservation Month—Come in for a Free Examination." It would be completely okay if the goal were to check out myopia. The problem develops when myopes with very low myopia (–0.25 or –0.50) are attracted by the advertisement and come to get their vision checked. They are immediately given "part-time" or "leisure" glasses to wear usually when watching TV or whenever they want to relax.

The result of this excessive sales pitch is that the myope, who could restore his normal refractive state quite easily at this threshold level through a functional rehabilitation program (learning the rules of sight hygiene, lessening the conditions of chronic stress, wearing positive lenses that could, rightly, be called "leisure" and "part-time glasses," or through short treatment with myopic defocus) is condemned to wearing "correcting" nega-

tive lenses whose dioptric power must be increased from time
to time.

- The health care culture typically does not deal with the issue of a
  patient who wants to be released from his symptom immediately
  without listening to the message his disease is "sending" him.

- We must open our eyes, listen to our disease, hear its message,
  and believe in our own power in healing our bodies, being led
  by treatments that are aimed at eliminating the causes of a
  problem and not just its symptoms.

What about Cinema?

Even the cinema was exploited by "booster commercials" on
Sight Preservation Month and when the *Harry Potter* book series
came out. Who was the star in the commercial on Sight Preservation Month? A boy wearing the same glasses as Harry Potter's.

Try to imagine what kind of subliminal, unnoticed message
could pass through innocent and naive children's and unaware
parents' minds: a "booster" to check their sight together with
instinctive childish emulation of Harry Potter's spectacled look.
Think it over folks . . . and please open your eyes.

The Reason Some Manage and Others Fail

If you are a personal trainer, you can reveal all the secrets and
the best techniques on athletic performance and muscular mass
increasing to your client, but it's up to her to *believe and trust* in
your instructions and suggestions and to *apply the techniques* in
doing the exercises.

She will be discouraged many times and then she'll need *trust*
and *perseverance:* it's like walking in the darkness and moving

toward the light—we have been told about how to do it, but we are unable even to imagine it.

As it has always been, only courageous people win: those who are endowed with great willpower and courage, perseverance, trust, and above all, who are ready to work hard to reach an important target within reason, logic, and facts. These people aren't satisfied with glib shortcuts, but go further, aware that they can get almost everything they wish in life if they understand the fundamental concept that the natural eye adapts its focal state to its visual environment.

Afterword

I often hear the words, "Prove it."

Since the "it" is never described, it follows that no one can ever "prove it." But David De Angelis has finally proven it—that it is possible to clear your distance vision. David's description is accurate, and the effort he has gone through suggests that your personal effort and resolve can produce successful results.

You will be surprised to know that a percentage of optometrists hold the same judgment, but they say that they cannot get most people motivated to do this work properly. Dr. Jacob Raphaelson identified this problem some time ago. The public wants its distance vision sharpened instantly and expects that all optometrists can do this. Anything beyond that point the public will reject—unless they are very intelligent and personally motivated about this difficult situation.

It is very clear that the person who desires prevention must have strong motivation and support from the optometrist. But the solution must start with your own willpower.

What are the difficulties of "recovery"? Mr. De Angelis and prevention-minded optometrists are clear on that point. The public demands immediate results and does not listen to explanations. Most people might quit an effort if there is the slightest problem or if another ophthalmologist or optometrist uses scare tactics against them. If this happens, they will quit the effort and blame the optometrist for anything that might happen with their eyes. There is scant incentive for optometrists to attempt to help the general public for that reason.

Many in the health professions judge that they have no choice but to apply a minus lens (with a few exceptions). This is tragic, because a large mass of scientific data tells us objectively that whenever the eye is placed in a "confined" environment it always moves in a negative direction—toward nearsightedness. This unfortunate situation has continued for a large number of years.

The theory of using a lens on the eye began this way:

1. The lens developers who were dealing with the public found a plus lens that would sharpen near vision—when you reached old age.

2. In addition, they found that young people with slightly blurry distance vision could instantly clear their distance vision with a minus lens.

The theory of using a lens is based on the traditional understanding of responsibility and the desire for direct action. There has been very little improvement in this concept. The theory that develops after the fact is used to explain away these bad results.

Around 1600, Johannes Kepler (an astronomer) began developing a pure refractive theory of the eye. This was good work, but assumed that you could "freeze" the eye and make all your measurements based on the box camera concept. This idea never attempted to analyze the eye's dynamic behavior at all—only the refractive properties of an intellectually frozen eye.

This analysis was good, so the fact that the eye is not frozen was forgotten. Kepler's analysis could be used to support Items 1 and 2. For this reason the "frozen eye" theory was accepted as a medical theory—and anyone who challenged the concept concerning the bad results of Item 2 were told that Kepler's theory was "proven" and that the natural eye is a rigid box camera.

Kepler's theory was further refined and republished in 1858 by two ophthalmologists, Dr. Donders and Dr. Helmholtz. They accepted Kepler's frozen-eye concept and added further assumptions.

1. They assumed that a focal state of exactly zero could be considered normal. Donders invented the word *emmetropia* to describe this idealization of the "frozen" eye.

2. They assumed that any focal state other than exactly zero must be a defect, or "refractive error." They invented the word *ametropia* to describe both positive and negative focal states of all normal eyes.

Don't get me wrong at this point: these were great men in medicine at that time. But they continued Kepler's academic assumption, that you could "freeze" the eye and do a pure refractive analysis. They also assumed that you could translate a relative focal state into an absolute dimension (that is, they assumed that if the eye had a focal state of zero, it must have an exact length of 24.38 mm. In fact, no relationship has ever been established).

By doing this, they thought that they had proved Kepler's theory that the eye was "too long," when the natural eye simply had a normal but undesired negative focal state.

This box camera theory made the use of a plus or minus lens seem more systematic, although it requires a belief that the eye is defective if it has a negative or positive focal state. (That is, if your eyes have a focal state that is not zero, you are suffering from "stress and strain" because the eye is too long or too short. The reasoning here is circular, because it is not proven that a focal state of zero corresponds to an exact length. It is only an assumption that you can convert relative measurements into absolute dimensions.) In any event, this theory makes all eyes defective by definition—a thesis of doubtful validity.

Why should we object to Kepler's theory, which became the theory of practice? As a theory that allows refractive analysis of an idealized eye, it is excellent. As a theory of the eye that reproduces the actual motion and change of focal state of the natural eye, it is not accurate. Kepler's pure refractive theory was correct, but the assumptions of the follow-up (Donders-Helmholtz) theory are not accurate or correct.

In light of experimental data developed in the past fifty years, we should begin developing a better conceptual model of the eye's dynamic behavior. The facts demonstrate that all eyes change their focal state as the visual environment is changed. The eye is established to be a well-designed autofocus camera (that is, you can make *all* eyes nearsighted by forced wearing of a minus lens).

The type of data needed to demonstrate this truth was not available in 1858. So the original concept should undergo evolution to account for these recently developed facts. But in fact, the operative reasons for using a plus or minus lens have not changed since their original inception four hundred years ago. Thus the "theory of the eye" is driven by expediency and not by objective scientific facts (in my humble opinion).

Science is based on objective facts. We should be able to recognize that there is a problem with expanding Kepler's theory beyond its original intended scope. He did an excellent refractive analysis. He did not intend that we believe that all eyes are rigid box cameras, that are defective because they have focal states other than zero.

We suggest that the natural eye is like an autofocus camera, and that, for this reason, the natural eye must change its focal state (which you measure) as you change the visual environment (which you control). Since we are using neutral language to describe this situation, it follows that experimental conformation (that all eyes are autofocus cameras) will be straightforward. This means that the evolution-designed eye can have both negative and positive focal states and not be defective.

In fact, the measured focal state of your eyes is directly dependent on your accommodation level, in diopters. Obviously, if you work for long hours, your normal eyes are going to develop a negative focal state. This is perfectly normal and expected for an autofocus camera.

The Helmholtz-Donders theory and its required assumption has never been objectively tested (as stated by Dr. William H. Bates). This means that the box camera image of the eye is misleading at best. At worst, it blinds us to a potential method of preventing the development of nearsightedness by aggressive use of a plus lens.

Diogenes searched the world over to find one honest man. We are continuing our quest for the answers that are important to you. To that end, we ask questions of science and experimental data that will help you to think through and get past potential roadblocks. We are considering some decidedly different possibilities about accommodation and the true long-term behavior of the eye. I believe that if we can come to a better working understanding of the visual system, you will be better able to prevent the eye's negative refractive change that we call "myopia."

—Otis Brown, author of *How to Avoid Nearsightedness*

Questions and Answers from the Power Vision System Website

I highly recommend that you carefully read this Questions and Answers section. You will gain a much deeper understanding of the Power Vision System techniques and you will find excellent suggestions for how to improve your vision training program and gain faster results.

If, after reading this section, you have further questions, please consult the support forum at www.powervisionforum.com.

1. *As you state it, this system looks miraculous.*
   Is it science or science fiction?

The Power Vision System (PVS) *isn't science fiction, but science.* The system is based upon the training of extrinsic ocular muscles, which are of the striated type, and therefore their physiological structure is equal to that of any other striated muscle in our body (like biceps or triceps). Also the ciliary muscle (smooth type, involuntary) could be efficiently trained with the visual biofeedback technique of the Accommotrac Vision Trainer. This is accomplished by wearing special training lenses and using the well-known concept of blur-driven accommodation. You can find such lenses easily at low cost, and they need be worn only during visual training work.

Ocular muscle training is based on the same principles as any other striated bodily muscle—the system just uses such principles and practices in a different way.

The principles are as follows:

a. The principle of gradual overloading

b. The SAID Principle (Specific Adaptation to the Imposed Demand)

2. *Who can guarantee me positive results from training with this method?*

This method is simply one of the methods, but it is *not* a magic pill. If you think you could learn something lying on the divan and watching TV instead of reading an interesting book—or improve your physical condition without "wasting" one single drop of sweat—this book and method will not work for you.

The Power Vision System is based on physiological laws and will work well for every single person (who suffers from hyperopic or myopic disorders) and at any age. However, personal commitment is required when using such physiological principles. If you are someone who wants everything (money, wealth, health) without investing time and effort, then this book will not work for you.

If you believe in *changes* and *possibilities* in your life, and the power of consciousness offers you the capability to improve and change your situation, then please use the principles of the Power Vision System with trust and perseverance.

3. *When I train while reading, I'm not able to make automatic focusing happen, despite the fact that I follow your instructions.*

There are two possible reasons:

a. Specifically, in the beginning of training with this method, the eyes are very weak because of low flexibility and strength and coordination of ocular muscles—a situation created while the person wore minus glasses. Over time, the glasses make the eyes "lazy," "freezing" natural and physiological focusing. The result is "stiff" eyes, which get tired easily. The solution for this problem is to carry out the Power Vision exercises of cyclorotation and fixation at the edges of visual field.

b. The other possible reason for your slow response is in automatic focusing. This could be due to an excessively long focusing distance for that training session. Remember that the load that is imposed on the eyes must lead to an adaptation; it shouldn't be excessive.

4. *When am I supposed to change my training glasses? When am I supposed to train with reading, focusing with higher dioptric power lenses on the training glasses?*

The right moment to change the lenses and wear higher dioptric power ones (for example, myopes from +1 to +2, and hyperopes from –1 to –2) is when the text is in focus while holding your reading material with completely extended arms and wearing your old training glasses.

The load—the lenses themselves—aren't a training load anymore because they aren't strong enough to create the slight "fogging" that is the most important and basic part of stimulating focusing. For hyperopes, when the text is in focus, at too short a distance, use a negative lens or an undercorrection and do defocus training at an higher distance.

The solution is to move to a higher dioptric power *training* lens.

5. *I'm not able to go further; my focusing looks as if it were steady at x distance.*

Focusing distance must be changed constantly throughout the time of training: the text must be moved to the *furthest* distance (for myopes) or at the *lowest* one (for hyperopes) so as to have an efficient stimulus for training by focusing constantly, and then, at that same distance, after opening your eyes widely for about 5 seconds and then blinking, you will notice you are able to focus well.

Focusing improvement doesn't always go continuously and gradually. You might not have any positive results even after two weeks of training. If you are focusing and carrying out ocular stretching correctly, *suddenly* you will notice remarkably better and clearer vision.

Keep trusting in the system and keep going with practice (solidifying the little improvements you have already achieved).

6. *Can I wear glasses and/or contact lenses and improve my sight at the same time?*

Wearing glasses with your current dioptric power prescription (or even worse, wearing contact lenses) could hinder the improvements in training with the Power Vision System. Wearing minus glasses (current dioptric prescription) is the *cause* of gradual sight deterioration; it is completely opposite to the Power Vision System concept. Training with the Power Vision System relaxes the state of chronic overaccommodation (which is mainly caused by constant near-work compounded by wearing minus glasses).

On the contrary, wearing corrective glasses causes a negative state of overaccommodation. Wearing minus lenses should be limited to conditions when they are absolutely needed (when required by the law—like driving vehicles, for instance). If you can't help wearing minus glasses (above all, in the case of high myopia), then it's advisable to wear undercorrection.

7. *I was told that not wearing glasses or contact (minus) lenses brings about sight deterioration.*

False! It's a mistaken myth that does nothing except make a billion-dollar business—money that goes into the pockets of the optical industry.

It's completely advisable to reduce a prescription (wherever possible for safety reasons) and limit wearing minus contact lenses and glasses. It's useful to repeat: Wearing contact lenses and glasses means greater visual stress, specifically in near-work, since this work stimulates visual processes that produce excessive accommodation and converging. This is the main reason that the eye's focal status moves in a negative direction and becomes nearsighted.

8. *I'm afraid of focusing when doing the exercises' ocular stretching. Could I damage my ocular muscles by forcing them too much?*

If you carry out the exercises correctly, with proper understanding of the principle of gradual, symmetric loading and at maximum range, you don't run any risk. It would be as if we could damage any bodily muscle by training it correctly.

Not only the body but also the mind responds to the change. Fears and doubts have a negative aim. By training ocular muscles, you can improve local blood circulation, which will bring about remarkable functional advantages.

9. *I feel some effects while carrying out ocular stretching and also after the training. What should I do?*

Whatever the muscular training, if it is carried out with untrained musculature, it can cause some discomfort. It means that you are overloading your eyes. Such *gradual* overloading will increase your eyes' performance, improving your sight and decreasing myopia.

10. *I don't have time to do the exercises.*

You can train your eyes at any moment throughout the day, and just a few rotations and symmetric movements are enough. You don't need to get your car and go to the gym, and neither do you have to shower after training.

11. *Where can I buy training glasses?*

At an optician's or at any other shop that is supplied with them. Don't waste your time explaining why you need them, because you could be laughed at or even persuaded that such glasses are "just an illusion." Demand your sight!

12. *Who is guaranteeing the final result of restoring clear, distant sight?*

Nothing is sure or guaranteed in our life. Nobody can guarantee your success. The only thing you can do is to trust in the method and persevere in doing the exercises, day after day.

13. *Does this method work well only for myopia or also for other visual disorders?*

My personal experience is with treating and healing myopia—but it doesn't mean that other visual disorders can't be treated with this restorative method.

The exercises of ocular stretching are surely useful and beneficial for training for focusing at a distance, but the very same principles can be used successfully even in the opposite way, for focusing at a near distance (as it happens with sight worsening). The only difference is this: we can use the same principles to improve our sight (gradual overload of focusing, either by moving the focusing point away for myopes or bringing it nearer for hyperopes) that are opposite to the reasons for sight deteriorating (both myopia and hyperopia—like constantly wearing glasses or contact lenses; too much near-work).

Obviously, everyone should carefully evaluate his or her own sight and its conditions and carry out the training program that is the most suitable. This is like a schedule for athletic training that must include the athlete's needs concerning his or her own bodily characteristics. The principles are the same, but they must be adjusted to one's personal needs.

However, I'm sure that even astigmatism could improve from ocular muscle training, since such training brings about a restoration of the balance between agonist and antagonistic ocular muscles.

14. *Does this method have anything to do with the Bates one?*

Dr. William Bates is surely a most important person for having turned our attention to the fact that the process of accommodation is closely linked with ocular muscles' perfect functioning, and that the shape of the eyeball can be modified by contracting and relaxing the extrinsic ocular muscles and changing focal point on the retina. (This is your refractive status, which is measured by using a trial lens kit (*phoroptor*) by you or your optometrist.)

Our method is different than the Bates Method, because in the Power Vision System the muscles are trained by using the two main features that rule muscular performance (here, focusing). These two factors are strength and flexibility. Bates insisted on a "light" approach of relaxing exercises (or movement). The Power Vision System insists on complete improvement of the most important characteristics and properties of ocular muscles: strength and flexibility.

To clarify, it's like the difference between (light) yoga and artistic gymnastics. The analogy is the situation where the athletes are trained well and their muscles are very flexible and strong. This is not by accident. The gymnasts are endowed with what's called "refined dexterity" in movements, which requires extremely precise coordination and motor qualities. Ocular muscles need this extraordinary quality—*refined dexterity*—to fulfill as complex a task as focusing is.

This phenomenon is underestimated, since we were born with this natural motor ability (in our eyes as well), but long, hard work is needed to become a gymnast. When you have a visual error, and you eventually reach 20/20 vision, your success is as though you obtained a 10/10 score at springboard. Surely, it's not an easy task. Undoubtedly the path to reach 20/20 exists, and the furrow has already been plowed, in my judgment.

15. *I have high myopia. As far as restoring my sight gradually and naturally, what are my chances of improving my situation since my present clinical state is the following: For eleven years my diopter has always been the same:*

Right Eye: 11.0 diopters   Astigmatism 1.5 at 180 degrees
Left Eye: 6.0 diopters   Astigmatism 1.0 at 180 degrees

Since last year, it has been:

Right Eye: 13.0 diopters   Astigmatism 1.0 at 125 degrees
Left Eye: 6.75 diopters   Astigmatism 1.75 at 165 degrees

But I still don't have a new pair of glasses.

As long as the technique is used correctly, this system works well. The limit is imposed by the person who trains with the system. When you notice the first visible (literally) improvements, you will easily understand that it's just a matter of practice.

It is true: the system requires great trust (in order to break one's own skepticism and achieve the first positive results). Just imagine yourself taking a degree in engineering (the commitment and effort required), but in this case your own eyes and your sight are on the scales.

I'll give you an example related to mechanical-architectural engineering to help you understand it more clearly. Understand the concept of *gradually* building (brick by brick) the difference between a middle-sized building and a castle. The first step depends on the worker's *engagement* (in our case, it depends on your commitment to doing the exercises, which are similar to the bricks) and on the *time* you spend in doing the exercises. Surely Rome wasn't built in a day, but I think, when dealing with a very important thing (like your vision), you must be very responsible and do it with great commitment.

In my example, I would be both the engineer and architect. The Power Vision System has established the ways of construction and I've checked them out by myself.

Do something for your eyes while you still have the time.

16. *I'm hyperope (+ 4 right eye, and + 4.50 left eye) and astigmatic. I kindly ask you to explain to me what your method would consist of in my case?*

Hyperopes have problems in focusing on near objects, since hyperopia is the opposite of myopia.

The Power Vision System is based on fundamental physiological principles, which are common to both refractive errors. (A positive refractive status is hyperopia and a negative refractive status is myopia.)

The most important and basic principle for the Power Vision System is the SAID Principle (Specific Adaptation to the Imposed Demand). This principle is well known in physiology (and in sports training); it means that the body has a natural ability to get used to induced stimuli.

Let's take an example from sports: an athlete who trains his or her muscles and physiological systems (for example, cardiovascular and respiratory systems) with induced loads in specific training. Such loads will cause a bodily response—an adaptation. In bodybuilding, for example, such a response is represented by anabolism, actually, by muscular hypertrophy.

In the case of treating refractive errors like myopia and hyperopia, the stimulus (the key factor for creating bodily adaptation, in this case of the eyes) must be *specific* and suitable for achieving the desired results. It's interesting to point out that such a stimulus must be *masterly* directed (so as to have positive results—recovery—and in our case, it means visual error regression until, in due course, a complete recovery). Otherwise, in the opposite case, it could cause the opposite results.

Now, you can see that every stimulus, badly imposed (directed) to the visual system, like wearing lenses or glasses in conditions when the eye could view correctly without them (for example, a hyperope who views distant objects wearing positive "correcting" lenses, ruins his own sight, causing *over*correction, which has negative effects on his proximal accommodation when he takes off his lenses). A completely opposite process works in case of myopia: a myope who wears glasses or contact lenses in near activities, worsens his refractive state furthermore, creating over-accommodation. When he takes off his glasses, his distance vision will be even worse.

The SAID Principle must have specific and differentiated use for each visual error, although it works well for both errors—myopia and hyperopia.

There's also a solution for your light exo/esophoria: to restore perfect ocular muscle symmetry through specific training of your extrinsic ocular muscles. Do you know that these little muscles are of the striated type and have the same structure as your biceps muscle (sarcomere: actine, myosine)? When you understand it, you'll be able to figure out that they have the same characteristics in training as any other bodily muscle. The laws are equal, but their use in practice is specific and different. The treatments should be directed, at first, to using *Natura Medicatrix* and natural laws before using any artificial means.

17. *I've already achieved improvements and stability in my vision. Will I be addicted to another therapeutic treatment? How do you check for muscular asymmetry? I completely understand the concept of doing the exercises and trust in the technique. Is it a matter of lifetime engagement (doing exercises for better accommodation) or is your technique the "resolute" one, through which, after a certain, necessary period of doing the exercises, a myope can restore his visual qualities, partially or completely, but permanently?*

The system gives permanent results, unless (so be careful) you subject your visual organs to those negative stimuli again (the stimuli that are ill omened for ocular accommodative capability).

Let me give you one simple and clear example: the myopes suffer from chronic *over*accommodation, due to near-work (functioning makes the organ and body get used to the imposed stimuli, both positive and negative [the SAID Principle]). According to these laws, you have been worsening your sight for years, wearing higher and higher negative dioptric power lenses. When you lessen this state of overaccommodation (until reaching the normal, clear, distinct sight—the emmetropic state), you must only follow and respect simple behavioral rules of "visual hygiene."

Obviously, if you put your minus glasses on again (with your ordinary dioptric power lenses), after having worked with the Power Vision System to relax the state of chronic overaccommodation, and then spend a long time in near-work activities, all the necessary conditions for creating myopia will be created again. The target is to give up certain negative habits and restore the balance of the extrinsic ocular muscles.

Without explaining the theoretical part completely, try this simple test that could help you become aware of your ocular muscles' asymmetry (imbalance between strength and flexibility, and consequently, coordination).

1. Stand in front of a mirror, and *without wearing your glasses* fix on the top of your nose. You must be as distant from mirror as permits you to see your nose well.

2. While maintaining binocular fixation, carry out symmetric movements of your face (for example, lower your chin, turn your head toward the right as much as you can, then toward the left as much as you can). Such movements (we can compare them to cardinal points) must be united into one *single* movement of head rotation, keeping fixed on your nose). The movements you carry out must be symmetric and without twisting. At a certain point, you'll eventually see the fixed image double (the top of your nose).

This means that your ocular muscles are asymmetric, and this condition reflects on *convergence* (the prevailing factor in myopia) as well as on the capability of focusing at Central Fovea (the most sensitive retinal part). The result: blurred vision due to the lack of the ocular muscles' coordination (are you able to keep fixing on a very fast object?) and due to the saccadic eye movement slowing down.

Your eyes should undergo specific rehabilitation with the specific exercises. The exercises proposed in this book are founded on physiological laws and you can find the sources in any scientific bibliography.

18. *From what I understand, your "method" is based on intelligent use of positive lenses for myopes and/or undercorrections. The lenses should have a different dioptric power in order to follow sight evolving, and the only problem I have at the movement is*

getting them. Am I supposed to buy an ophthalmologic kit, or is
it better to have a new pair of glasses made from time by time?

No ophthalmologic kit.

You can easily find the glasses you need at a pharmacy or drug
store but also at large stores like K-Mart or Wal-Mart (at $10 to
$15). You'll need glasses +1, +2, and +3 (if you're myopic). The
combination of these lenses (for example, +3 with +2) will lead
you forward in your training by increasing the stimulus. Later on,
when you reach a higher level, you can add +4 lenses, creating +7
stimulus together with +3 lenses. You can buy such glasses at a low
price—*much* lower than for a pair of ordinary minus-prescription
glasses, which cost $100 or higher.

Training with such glasses will lead you to throw away your
glasses *forever* (no matter what kind you are wearing at the
moment) and, even in the worst case, to improving your sight a
great deal. It depends on *your* practicing with commitment. The
method and means (actually the technique) does exist!

19. *I'm a bit of a skeptic. I've been doing the exercises. I was taught*
by a therapist. I started 15 months ago (I wore contact lenses
–4.75 and –4.50) and now I wear –2.25 and –2.00 ones. My
recovery has been going very slowly, but it does goes on. Now I'm
doing it by myself, repeating a few exercises that my teacher has
taught me. I think it's not the Bates Method, because I've read
many books on the issue and I know that the Bates Method is
based on relaxation. I desperately want to see well without the
help of any means. I've spent a lot of money on glasses, contact
lenses, liquids, therapeutic sessions.

I've always been interested in learning—above all else—what
I need. I would also like to speed up my sight improvment (if

possible). I'm very interested in all that you say, but I am a skeptic about buying something without having examples of its effectiveness. Please give me some examples of your method so I can decide whether to buy it or not.

Being interested in learning and knowing more has caused me to purchase many a rip-off. Once I bought a book on "visual reeducation" for $25. Twenty-five dollars for twelve pages! Using the same metric, the Power Vision System should be offered at a substantially higher price.

I think you are going in the right direction, since you've improved your sight so remarkably. I think your trainer is excellent.

As I've written, my system is based on:

a. Using the lenses of *opposite* dioptric power to the ordinarily worn ones (for example, myopes should wear *positive* instead of *negative* lenses). Such a system acts on the ciliary muscle's overaccommodative state. *Keep in mind:* There's a specific way to graft focusing (normally it is an automatic process. The system is called ocular CRB movement).

b. Increasing coordination and ocular mobility. Do this simple test: Fix your vision at the top of your nose, standing in front of a mirror at 3 feet distance (if you are able to see your nose well from that distance, otherwise come nearer to the mirror). Carry out symmetric rotations at the maximum range of ocular movement, turning your face (for example, as far up as you can, toward the left, toward the right, always as much as you can) while fixing on your nose.

You will see that in some parts of your visual field (if the movements are symmetric and at maximum range), the image will become double (or, at least, you'll have trouble maintaining a fusion of the fixed point, in this case of your nose).

It means that point b, through the exercise of muscular working at *maximum* range, will lead you to remarkably better fusion, which is needed—and is basic for perfect focusing, since the image must fall on the central fovea (the most sensitive retinal part); otherwise it would be blurred (it depends on how far from the central fovea the image falls).

Keep going on this way, and trust in what you're doing. When you see well again, not only will you *see* clearly, but you'll also be aware of having done something really special in your life and you'll *understand* that everything is possible if you believe you can get it.

20. *I tried the Accommotrac, getting some good results, but not as good as I expected. I'm a myope at –0.75 D in my right eye and –1.25 D in my left eye. Why should your method work better than the Accommotrac? I've also read Bates. I never wear glasses, and my sight hasn't worsened a lot in these years, despite the fact that I've been working at computer a lot.*

I'll do my best to explain to you about Accommotrac Vision Trainer limits—and why PVS works well.

The eyes must point at central parts of the visual field in training with Accommotrac: your gaze must be directed and "blocked" toward ahead. This very thing happens while wearing glasses, but then, the eyes are not "stimulated" to view at the limits of ocular movement range, which is much wider than the ordinary one used when wearing glasses. This kind of functioning is abnormal, and, with time, it jeopardizes the extrinsic ocular muscles' functioning.

Your ocular capability is characterized by involuntary ocular movements that are extremely fast—so called saccadic movements. When basic ocular endowments become weak because of working at a limited range (as it happens wearing glasses or in training with Accommotrac), the eyes gradually lose their full saccadic movements' functioning and, consequently, their focusing ability.

The Accommotrac works well, but it has its own limits, which could be overcome by supplementing it with the techniques as described in PVS.

I think it's important to point out that training by use of a focusing machine could be replaced with a system that isn't based on sound but on proper visual biofeedback. The latter system consists of a clever use of the lenses that are opposite to the visual error (if you're a myope you should train wearing the lenses for hyperopes or train with undercorrected glasses). However, nothing could be improved by the simple wearing of the opposite lenses because there is a very precise technique to be followed.

The most important thing is personal commitment and effort in carrying out the Power Vision System technique for some time. We should remember the principle: Knowledge is worthless unless you use it.

21. *What is your advice for using training lenses? What dioptric power should I start with? I have myopia and strabismus. My right eye is –6 ast. and my left one is –6.25 ast. –2.25.*

   a. *Where could I buy training lenses? Are they the kind I can find for $15 to $30 in the stores?*

   b. *What dioptric power I should start with?*

   c. *Are the training lenses to be used in addition to my present correction or apart?*

   d. *Am I supposed to feel some muscular "stiffness" in order to see that the CRB movement exercise is carried out correctly?*

You are quite lucky since your myopia is almost equal in both your eyes.

   a. You can find the glasses you need at an optician's, drug store, or in most large stores.

   b. and c. As for dioptric power, you should be able to train with reading a book or newspaper, creating a state of *slight* fogging. Try to create it without lenses, while reading. Try to move the book away from your eyes until you create this slight fogging. Then, carry out the CRB movements, and, in the end, blink, to relax your eyes.

Important: You must create a certain, basic ocular strength and flexibility through stretching at maximum ocular range.

At the beginning, your self-focusing system (now "frozen" because of wearing glasses and contact lenses for years) will be reluctant to work, but trust and believe in the system and keep going on.

At a certain point you will see that after CRB movements all that was previously blurred now becomes clear. When you understand this principle, everything will be only a matter of great patience and perseverance.

The eyes get used to the lenses with time, and therefore you must increase the stimulus (either moving the text away or increasing dioptric power of your training lenses).

   d. The feeling of this "work" is very personal. However, by opening your eyes wide, you will feel some eye stiffness.

You must try several times, changing your lenses until you find the most suitable ones. Start without lenses (if you can) or wear your present glasses with another additional pair over, with positive lenses +1 and +2. You must create fogging before carrying out CRB movements.

22. *I'm thirty now and probably the "shape" of my eye (if hyperopia depends on the shorter eye) can't be modified a lot, at least, not as much as in childhood: is this true or false? Despite the present boom of refractive surgery and the associated billion-dollar business, I'm suspicious about such methods. I'm a hyperope with +4.5 for my left eye and 20/20 in my right eye. Lately I've been thinking of starting to wear a blindfold over my right eye to force the left one; as once, a long time ago, I was ordered to do so by an oculist—but probably the " shape" of my eye can't be modified as much as it could be in childhood.*

Is it possible by practicing with your method that we can get positive results? Is there any limit for practicing your method at an "elderly" age?

Just one question more—but I wouldn't like you to misunderstand it: Why do you want to sell me your book, if you are pushed by so great a praiseworthy and altruistic desire to spread and share your discovery and your knowledge?

I can understand your doubts completely.

You say, "I'm thirty now and probably the 'shape' of my eye can't be modified as much as in childhood. . . . "

I ask, Who has said that? What kind of science is that statement based on? Who has ever stated that muscular tissue can't be modified or get used to suitable stimulus through specific exercises?

People who deal with such issues professionally have no time to explain to you certain things (if they even know about them). Sometimes it's easier to put a pair of glasses onto someone's nose than to spend time explaining and above all teaching you about this method. Usually, the person who checks your sight also sells glasses, and not everybody is ready to work their way out of their visual defect: they prefer to accept the opinion that nothing can be done to resolve refractive errors. Everybody is free to choose what he wants and likes, even though it may only be a temporary "quick fix."

Age doesn't make any difference for getting positive results in working with the system: PVS is based on physiological concepts that work well at any age. As long as you are able to "command" and control your ocular movement, you'll also be able to restore your ocular symmetry and consequently your "central fixation"— which is fundamental for clear, distinct vision.

23. *I have some questions on the exercises:*

    a. *Does your method work well for strabismus (esotropia or exotropia)?*

    b. *Should the rotations in stretching be slow or fast? For how long a time am I supposed to hold onto a certain position in stretching without rotations?*

    c. *In the advanced training program, does "twice" (in the exercises) mean that I must put my eyes in a certain position two times?*

    d. *Dioptric power between my left and right eye is 1.5 grades (0.50 and 2.00). I've found out that my better eye views for the "bad" one and that the latter is getting lazy. Since I think it's hard to bring both eyes to the same visual acuity, do I run any risk of having one of my eyes idle, which would become lazy with time and consequently would bring about ocular defect worsening? As for training for focusing—could it be carried out with only one eye (the lazy one), covering the other?*

    e. *I read about a guy whose myopia was very high, but he decided not to wear lenses and his sight improved (despite your statement there's no adapting without fogging). What do you think about this story? If I gave up everything, became a farmer, and did no exercises, wouldn't my sight improve? Then if I went on a mountain to view the landscape, wouldn't my ocular acuity improve?*

The system works well for focusing and, above all, it works completely. The exercises provide high ocular coordination and a gradual restoration of focusing.

I've tested the system by myself and I've had great results—I've defeated my myopia. Therefore the system surely works well also for hyperopes, considering that the means of intervening are the same: increasing the ocular ability of placing the image on the most sensitive retinal part—the central fovea—together with the clever use of training lenses.

a. As for your strabismus, I can't guarantee its complete healing since I don't have complete evidence or proof. It does not mean that the system couldn't work for decreasing the strabismus gradually: including better oculomotor muscle functioning (extrinsic ocular muscles) together with resultant better focusing that are likely to bring about astigmatism decreasing, at least indirectly. But I can't guarantee it. It's up to you—the reader—to prove and confirm such a hypothesis, trusting and practicing in the method.

b. The speed in doing the exercises of ocular stretching should be slow and controlled. Such kind of stretching is called "active static stretching." Ocular muscles' lengthening and stretching happens, in a certain portion of visual range, by means of *agonist* (contracting) muscle and its *antagonistic* (lengthening/extending) muscle. Every muscle could be both agonist and antagonist, depending on a movement it's carrying out at that very moment.

When you look down, some of your ocular muscles are agonist, and the others, which are placed in the opposite ocular section, are antagonist. In the opposite case, when you look down, the exact opposite thing will occur. This "stretching out" is caused by shortening and contracting the opposite muscle (strengthening); therefore the muscles are to be contracted with a certain intensity.

Use rotations and slow, controlled "pointing," focusing on those parts of visual field where it's harder to carry them out and where we feel a "block" or a trough movement (such phenomenon proves the importance and the need for restoring exact local muscular symmetry to bring about more precise pointing and focusing).

c. I meant full rotations—the entire turn each one: two rotations with your eyes opened and two with closed eyes. The purpose is a kind of "warming up" for your ocular muscles so as to make them ready for further exercises. Training protocols depict the standard way. You are allowed to adjust them to your own needs. For example, if in one part of your ocular range you notice double vision, which reveals muscular asymmetry, you must stay in that very portion of visual range. The training routine in PVS is aimed at creating possible ways of working with higher and higher intensity. A period of time is needed for whatever kind of training you carry out, so that you can do it easily—even at the advanced level.

d. Your fear is reasonable. The difference in focusing ability between your two eyes tends to prevail for the "better" eye's vision. The final result is that your brain tends to use the perception of the more healthy eye, gradually making lazy and worsening the less capable one.

A solution exists: to first train the eye that suffers from a greater visual defect—by blindfolding your "better" eye. Your ability in focusing will gradually improve with this procedure—and little by little, each will become equal to the other eye's focus. Only at that point can you train both your eyes together at the same time.

Such a procedure is aimed at avoiding suppression of the "worse" eye and consequently the possibility of its becoming lazy. However, you'll have great advantages and positive results from this work.

e. Many famous and important authors (like Aldous Huxley and William Bates) have proved to themselves and their patients a better focusing ability.

All that has been proved about sight clearing after giving up the wearing of corrective lenses and living "in the open air" isn't a secret, and it is proven in many studies on near-point stress (due to overaccommodation) and behavioral reasons for myopia. The seminal study carried out with Eskimo families was by Francis A. Young (1969), titled "The Transmission of Refractive Errors within Eskimos Families." The fogging during the exercises of focusing with the lenses on *must* be light, otherwise our brain would consider focusing an impossible duty and consequently wouldn't even try to do it. I'm referring to the phenomenon of blur-driven accommodation. It's true that when you are outdoors and have less near-point stress (overaccommodation), your sight (refractive status) will get better. This has nothing to do with the importance of the training stimulus that must be imposed on the visual system and it is needed to achieve focusing system adaptation. Both living in the open air and slight fogging are needed to induce a "positive" adaptation of focusing system and resultant distance vision clearing.

24. *When I'm able to focus a text well, holding it with completely extended arms, does this mean that I'm supposed to change my plus lenses? For how long a time should each stretching position be maintained while carrying out the exercise of stretching (in seconds)?*

a. *Starting from focusing: I put my glasses on (I always wear under-correction, when studying or working) and then I put a +1 additional lens over my correcting lenses, move the book as far away in order for the letters to be slightly blurred, carry out CRB movements, stretching out my eyes and eyebrows as much as I can and have the letters come into focus—even if not perfectly. Am I right? Then, I take off the +1 additional lens while blinking, wait for some seconds, put the +1 additional lens back, move the text away until the letters are slightly blurred, carry out the CRB movements and so on. Am I carrying it out correctly?*

b. *Am I supposed to keep my gaze fixed on certain details or I can space it over the page?*

c. *Should I change the plus additional lenses once I'm able to focus the text well, holding it in completely extended hands?*

d. *Passing to static gymnastic: I take off my glasses, because I can't focus anything well if I wear my glasses, and carry out the exercises at extreme positions of the visual field; one of my eyes views through the lens, but the other doesn't.*

e. *When fixing on a point and turning my head till maximum ocular tension (for example, toward the left, as much as possible), at a certain point my right eye vision is completely, or partially, covered with my nose: is it okay, or too much?*

f. *For how long am I supposed to keep in one stretching position (as well as all the positions in the exercises of stretching), in seconds?*

I'm pleased and willing to answer all your questions:

a. The sequence you are carrying out is correct and there's no need to take off the additional lenses (+1 in your case, but dioptric power of the additional lenses would be +2, +3, +4, at a higher stage in practicing this technique, or if you were treating hyperopia, the lenses would be negative). On the other hand, if your myopia were low, you could train with training lenses even without putting them over your ordinary, correcting glasses, wearing only training lenses. The explanation for the latter is that your myopia is low (about 2 diopters per eye), the fogging (driven for reading the text) is "reasonable," even without your present dioptric power glasses.

As reasonable, I mean the method or technique that lets you create slight fogging and focus on the text without holding it 3–4 inches from your nose (as you should do if your myopia were high and if you immediately trained without your ordinary lenses but with the opposite sign). As for high myopia, it is necessary to put the training lenses over the ordinary ones; then, as your focusing is improving, you take off your ordinary lenses and/or even increase the dioptric power of your training lenses. The adaptation is inevitable, otherwise we wouldn't be able to explain gradual sight worsening.

You don't need to take off your training glasses after CBR movements.

b. The gaze can move all over the paper, but if you want to read the text you are training with, you must "point" the line and the letters you would like to focus on, as when reading normally.

c. Yes, but it's a matter of convenience. When you reach the stage of training with reading, wearing additional +1 lenses, and holding the text in completely extended arms, you must change the lenses and use higher dioptric power training ones, simply because, otherwise, it would be hard to read the text at a further distance.

The simplest thing to do is to increase the training load for your eyes, putting higher dioptric power training lenses over the others. Now you can see that the length of your completely extended arms that you take as a limit for the present training lenses is a matter of convenience and, therefore, the sign to change them.

Keep in mind: In the case of hyperopia, the text should be brought nearer gradually—and the training lenses could be changed for higher dioptric power ones (passing from –1 to –2 and then to –3, concerning your refractive error). When you bring the text too close to your nose, there's *no* slight blur: then, since the load doesn't exist anymore (because your eye has gotten used to training lenses, improving its focusing ability), it will be necessary to rebuild the load with higher dioptric power lenses (the training ones).

d. Yes, you must take off your glasses when carrying out the exercises of ocular stretching; otherwise these glasses would hinder your peripheral fusion and pointing. At this early stage, you must maintain ocular fusion (opposite to splitting). This is the aim of these exercises—to restore the symmetry (flexibility/strength ratio) of extrinsic ocular muscles. In short, maintain the fusion of the fixed point at the edges of the visual field.

e. Your nose shouldn't jeopardize your training, and you must stop your glance before one of your eyes becomes covered with your nose; otherwise you can't tell whether your eyes are in the state of fusion or splitting.

f. I need to explain some concepts on contraction intensity and muscular work. As for muscular work, the intensity is the relationship between *quantity of load* that is moved in a *time* unit. In the case of isometric contractions (when the muscle is contracting against a steady resistance), and in our case, it is impossible to give you precise suggestions on the factor of contraction intensity.

How can we avoid this merely theoretical factor? How can we be sure that our eyes are always subjected to the load that is suitable to create muscular adaptation? The answer is in perceiving the level of muscular work you are carrying out. Muscular work (the intensity of contraction) depends on your willingness: you must fix at the extreme point of your visual field as if you wanted to overcome that very range of movement.

The time? 10 seconds or 1 minute—it depends on how much muscular work you would like to carry out. The greater the intensity, the more you bring about muscular recovery—strength increase and better ocular muscles' functioning.

Don't worry if you didn't understand some of these technical explanations. You aren't supposed to understand cardiovascular circulation functioning in order to make your heart work. All that you are supposed to do is to use and practice the technique.

25. *How about it: you state that we shouldn't wear special lenses more than 2 hours per day (in the intense program)! Why?*

The answer to your question is in the capability of our body to get used to different, induced stimuli: Exposing any physiological system to specifically and systematically repeated stimuli inevitably leads to changes in the that organ's functioning. Regarding focusing, it means that specific exercises lead to modifications and consequent positive changes in focusing.

So as to trigger the body's capability of getting used to the induced stimuli, we need a stimulus of certain intensity, which could be empirically quantified as training time.

Following the technique correctly, the most important factor is to calibrate the stimulus intensity so as to ensure it will be enough to trigger the adaptation without being excessive and therefore "unproductive." It's completely useless to overcome the adaptation threshold of any physiological system; therefore, it would be useless if someone trained with training lenses or did the exercises of ocular stretching for 24 hours. You can't achieve improvements, since the body (and mind) have to take their own time for this adjustment or change to take place.

Imagine an athlete who is lifting weights and wants to increase his strength and muscular mass. He would practice according to his own training program for strength increase, lifting heavier and heavier weights (intensity—otherwise, after a while, it wouldn't be a training stimulus at all). If he trained for 3 hours a day or 8 hours a day, his performance wouldn't increase; excessive stimulus could even be self-defeating, jeopardizing recovery and body adjustment.

I've set up a 2-hours-daily training limit for the advanced program, since it's estimated as a maximum stimulus to achieve the improvements fast and without jeopardizing your focusing ability.

The eyes need a maximum stimulus that is both suitable for training and also creates positive adaptation, like a positive focus change. The body needs time to get used to the exercises, as does your mind, which needs time to get used to perceiving the world that now appears clearer and with enhanced shadings.

The visual process isn't merely a physiological one, but one that involves deeper parts of the human psyche and our relationship with ourselves and with others. The way we relate to ourselves is with respect to our mind. Am I not said to be myopic-minded? The body is the soul's mirror: when you understand it you will also understand how to work on your body. Your mental and emotional horizons are widening toward spiritual and holistic healing—and this involves all the states of "being" and not only the physical ones.

26. *How long will it take to recover from my 4.5 D in my left eye?*
   How long did it take you to recover?

Nobody can tell you in exact terms the time needed to restore your focusing ability; it's also very hard to estimate it, since it depends on many factors—your initial refractive state, the kind of work you are doing, your visual environment, and the kind of effort you are willing to make. Also included is time you spend using your "protective" lenses and your personal verification of results by checking your own eye chart.

I can say that the time you need to improve your sight depends on the quantity of your training and, above all else, on wearing your "preventive" glasses.

Let me explain further: if someone trains 5 minutes a day and someone else trains for 20 minutes, obviously the time they need to reach the flashes of distinct, clear vision is different. It's useless to do the exercises and then spend all the day at a computer, wearing your minus glasses, because in such a case overaccommodative stress (proximal stress produced by the minus lens) persists. One thing is certain: the time needed to get improvements is much shorter than the time it took to worsen your sight (which induced your present dioptric prescription).

Being supervised by an optometrist or an ophthalmologist, you can start to do cyclorotations: slow and concentrated on the present maximum range of your eyes, and symmetric. Later on, you can start doing the exercises on retinal defocus so as to bring about a better refractive state. As for this, you should take advice from your physician.

27. *Why does it take less time to achieve better visual acuity with*
   the Power Vision System than to notice sight worsening, that is,
   wearing minus lenses for myopes?

You can expect faster improvement in such cases if the program of sight rehabilitation is carried out correctly: at first acting over muscular properties and the symmetry of oculomotor muscles, and later on over suitable retinal defocus, constantly following the rules of visual hygiene. In such case, the improvements are faster than when wearing minus lenses for myopes, because of wrong use of hyperopic retinal defocus.

When we are subjected to overaccommodative stress and defocus negative stimuli, wearing glasses with minus lenses causes your eyes to adjust toward counterbalancing/compensating for hyperopic defocus. (This also happens when a myope views near while wearing full negative correction.)

With the Power Vision System, the refractive (defocus) stimuli don't happen by chance. Once aware of the effect of negative stimuli on your refractive ability, you should do your best to lessen the overaccommodative stress (either by wearing undercorrection or plus lenses), or you should work directly with myopic retinal defocus in the case of myopia.

Chance stimulation leads to slow adaptation, because the stimuli are directed without being aware of the reason. Being aware of stimulating our refractive system, as happens in the Power Vision System, lets us achieve positive results much faster, because the more we are aware of stimuli and induce them voluntarily, the more often they are repeated. At the same time, we should lessen and consciously avoid negative stimuli (overaccommodative stress). The sum of such stimulating leads to adaptation and consequently to refractive change.

28. *About the issue of restoring and improving the extrinsic ocular muscles' coordination and central fixation/centralization, I'm following the Power Vision System and I'm getting much better:*

still 2 diopters per each eye, maybe at the moment just 1.5 thanks to the exercises you've proposed in your book.

I still have one problem I'm not able to resolve. When I look up, I notice that my right eye stops before the left one, and they don't converge equally. Should I continue doing the exercises, looking up, till the extrinsic muscles around my right eye get relaxed, therefore becoming able to extend as much as the left eye's muscles? Do you have any other exercise I can use for my right eye?

A healthy eye is perfectly able to point/fix at an observed object in all the parts of the visual field (both in the central parts and the extreme ones—as when you look up or aside as much as you can). Perfect ocular coordination is the result of the extrinsic ocular muscles' perfect functioning. After being rehabilitated, from the point of view of functioning, through different specific exercises (rotation and movement), the oculomotor muscles also restore their flexibility, strength, and consequently coordination between the right and the left eye that allows your eyes to do the work that is required for correct focusing.

Don't forget that a healthy eye has a capability of "vibrating," which is characterized by saccadic movements and a pointing/fixating ability at all levels of ocular movement and in all parts of the visual field, including the peripheral ones, which are not used when wearing glasses. Even visibly, when observing healthy eyes, you can notice a different ability of viewing. The eyes that suffer from high myopia have an almost missing gaze, without fixing at anything: indeed it's so, since myopes have a very low ability of achieving central fixation (some authors call this ability "centralization").

Centralization or central fixation is the ocular ability of making the image fall on the central fovea. If the extrinsic ocular muscles are not well coordinated (because of low strength and flexibility at the edges of visual field), just one or both eyes make the image converge and fall out of central fovea—on the yellow spot (*macula lutea*).

The phenomenon is called "retinal eccentricity"; it is also responsible for low focusing ability. When the eyes get back their ability of coordinating (and there are some exercises like ocular rotations and their variants that bring about better coordination), they will also be able to point and focus correctly on the central fovea again. Furthermore, the eyes will also start to vibrate perfectly again, having restored their normal saccadic movement.

Sometimes, certain anomalies in coordinating are possible during muscular rehabilitation through the exercises of rotation (especially in rotation fixing at a point). It's necessary to restore perfect coordination, staying in the parts where you feel the "knots," when the eyes aren't able to maintain binocular fixation (fixing at a point while rotating), which results in double vision. These results show the problem of coordination between the eyes as well as your ocular symmetry imbalance. Little by little, persist on rotating while fixing at a point in those parts of the visual field where you have some problems in coordinating/fixing, and you'll notice better coordination/fixation and consequently better visual acuity.

The extrinsic ocular muscles are the striated type and, therefore, are subject to the same rules of "plasticity" and adaptation as any other striated muscle of our body (biceps, triceps). So, it's necessary to train the ocular muscles according to one's specific needs and then to go further with the exercises of retinal defocus, as described in the Power Vision System. *Keep in mind:* At first the exercises apply for muscular rehabilitation (like rotations), and the exercises of retinal defocus come later (with or without training lenses). Before learning to run, your muscles must walk.

29. *Is the Power Vision System based on any scientific elements? How did you figure it out? Please, let me know how and where could I get it. . . . I did some exercises with a therapist for two years, and I had some small improvements (from –5 to –2.5 D), but then I gave up practicing because I was fed up, and probably my sight got worse. I work at computer a lot and my job requires a lot of near-work.*

The Power Vision System is based on physiological reactions like SAID (Specific Adaptation to the Imposed Demand) or retinal defocus, which have important and proven effects on the human body. The SAID Principle concerns gradual bodily adaptation to specifically induced stimuli, which leads to functional and structural changes in the treated organ—in this case, the eyes and the visual system.

The principle of retinal defocus concerns focusing-system compensation or adaptation to the induced stimulus: in the case of myopia a person is subjected to myopic defocus (becoming more myopic, lessening dioptric power of his lenses, or in case of middle/low myopia wearing positive training lenses). Such a phenomenon is called "fogging" and represents a "trigger"—the stimulus for retinal compensation. The training is aimed at using retinal defocus/fogging masterfully and specifically for each and every case of myopia/hyperopia.

The Power Vision System could also be considered a scientific method, since it's based on physiological laws that are ascertained by traditional science. In addition, the effects of retinal defocus have been ascertained in studies on animals and especially in primates/monkeys.

If by *scientific* you are asking whether the Power Vision System was tested and the results were published in the journals on optometry, I can inform you that such tests haven't been done yet. They are likely to be tested in humans soon.

A new scientific and experimental thesis is never born together with a series of studies and experiments proving it; otherwise it wouldn't be new or experimental. This process of scientific understanding, and the results of scientific experiments, are described in Thomas Kuhn's book, *The Structure of Scientific Revolutions* (1996; 3rd ed.).

The Power Vision System has been written to explain and detail a system of treatment concerning both the physiological laws that it is based on as well as psychological phenomena beyond the visual system, such as bioenergetics. The system has worked in my case, but it's up to each of us to check out its validity—taking upon ourselves the responsibility while being supervised by an oculist or an optometrist.

If you want to see whether this system works, you need to do the following: try to feel the effects of myopic retinal defocus without wearing contact lenses or glasses for half a day (you must be at a safe place, where you aren't supposed to wear full correction for your personal or others' safety). You are likely to notice or, at least, to have impressions of, better visual acuity at the end of the experiment: such improvement is a direct consequence of the visual system adapting to retinal defocus.

The Power Vision System acts directly and gradually, stimulating the visual system, getting used to and aiming at gradual regressing of functional visual error. Since the error is functional, the problem should be resolved by acting over working ability: this is the basis of visual reeducation.

You say you're working at a computer, being obliged to view near, and you've also noticed that your sight has gotten worse after some positive results you achieved while working with your (very good) therapist. This phenomenon is due to the fact that you are constantly subjected to overaccommodative stress and constant visual axis' converging (the latter needs the process of accommodation to act). If you want to keep all the positive results you have reached, you must allow your eyes to "space" over long distances. In doing so, the tonic accommodation will relax and the ocular axis will become parallel (eliminating the stimulus for converging).

As a preventive measure, you can also wear undercorrection (or a plus lens) when working at the computer. It is enough to wear undercorrection whenever you carry out near-distance activities or to lessen the accommodation through positive lenses. In the end, I would like to tell you that it works—really works! Certifications, diplomas, and scientific studies aren't needed to ascertain something from our own experience. Work with the Power Vision System while being supervised by a physician, optometrist, or ophthalmologist.

30. *Help! My sight is getting worse and worse. How could I avoid harming my sight for the rest of my life? I've been a myope for some years (0.25—0.50 D per each eye). Once I had perfect sight and I'm very sorry I can't see as well as before. I study and work at the same time. Does this "work" somehow bring about my sight getting worse? I need clear, distinct sight for my job.*

It's very interesting to notice (and point out) your gradual development of almost all functional visual errors. If you ask anyone who suffers from a refractive error, he is likely to answer, "At the moment I wear –4 diopters, but at the beginning, my first pair of glasses was –0.75" referring to gradual dioptric power change in a negative direction.

Analyzing these simple answers, we can see that each person was changing her glasses constantly throughout the time due to her sight getting worse. It makes us wonder whether the "corrective procedure" works well from a therapeutic point of view, since in almost all cases it doesn't cure the very problem at all, but even worse, it is contributing to the increase of overaccommodative/near-point stress. This results in decreasing focusing ability over time.

In recent years, medical science has made great steps and presently can treat a huge number of diseases and problems, but in this case of functional visual disorders we should wonder: What has been done for accommodative functional disorders like myopia, hyperopia, or astigmatism? Could we see the indiscriminate wearing of minus glasses and contact lenses as a therapeutic procedure?

Perhaps the present "treatments" for refractive errors should be checked out again from another point of view, which must be less "myopic," knowing about the importance of the need for effective prevention. When someone's leg is broken, the first step is to put it in a cast in order to heal the bone. Such a procedure is aimed at allowing the injured person to walk on his legs again. Sometimes he's also given a pair of crutches to support his body weight and to make walking easier, until his leg is completely healed and the injured person is able to walk again. *Keep in mind:* The crutches are to be used until the leg is healed and walking is restored—but not beyond that point.

This does not happen in healing the sight by prescribing and wearing minus-lens glasses. Try to imagine a person who goes through a bad time and notices that his sight is getting worse. The person has a feeling of not being able to see well, and that what he could previously see is now blurry. Therefore, he looks for an ophthalmologist who diagnoses him as having low myopia and "heals" him with a pair of minus-lens glasses.

From this moment on, wearing such glasses, even at "near" where he doesn't need them at all, this person's refractive error will be getting worse and worse. A "functional error" is one that doesn't act over the structure of an organ (organic disease) but over the way the organ is used—in this case, wearing minus glasses, or even worse, wearing full correction contact lenses (20/20—Snellen chart, per each eye) over time. When you do this, the visual system will become weak and tired (consequently, higher and higher dioptric power minus lenses will be needed). In my view, this can't be the right therapeutic procedure, since it doesn't remove the initial cause of problem itself, but worsens it over time.

So, we shouldn't be surprised when we notice that a person who wears full correction in almost all his ordinary activities demonstrates this myopic "propensity" and gradual sight worsening. This type of "minus-lens therapeutic" procedure for refractive errors degenerates the optically overcorrected person into an endless series of newer and stronger minus-lens glasses. The result: Growing older, the refractive error will, most probably, grow.

The rule "Function makes the organ" doesn't foresee any exception even in the case of visual organs; natural and physiological focusing ability becomes worse and is "ruined" by wearing full correction (minus glasses and contact lenses), as we do presently. Besides, such a procedure does not act on someone's personal psychological, emotional, or other additional causes, nor on the stress itself.

Perhaps the reader is under too high overaccommodative stress (working and studying a lot). She might be under other kinds of stress at the same time (remember that the eyes suffer from emotional stress more than other organs), and all this has led to her sight going more negative. However, it could be healed in this initial phase simply by lessening the near-point/proximal stress (viewing in distance and, perhaps, wearing positive "leisure" glasses for all near-work). Besides, it would be very useful to have some break in your ordinary activities and to let yourself relax and rest. If you decide to wear positive lenses, it will reduce near-point stress and will improve distance focusing ability. However, you are to wear such plus lenses only when you don't need full distant correction for safety reasons (for example, driving your car or doing a particular job).

31. *I've been doing the exercises for over a year and half, looking for healing hyperopia in my left eye, blindfolding my right eye, and carrying out "slow" rotations with my left eye, as you recommended. I've got some positive results, but I don't know how much my hyperopia has decreased (I started with about 4 diopters). Unfortunately, lately I haven't noticed the same improvements as before. Shall I ever be able to eliminate my problem completely and have 20/20 sight? If I blindfold my right eye so as to make the left one work more, why do I need a lens to "worsen" my focusing?*

    Since there's already a defect, I believe that the eye should try, by itself, to focus an image correctly until getting back to normal 20/20. That's the reason I'm not able to understand what the lens is needed for, since it makes the image even more out of focus.

    As for "the flashes of clear vision" you talk about, I have had just two of them, usually at night, and later on, I noticed a clear improvement. It happened some time ago and now—nothing, as if everything stopped, just a few, slight "stretching" feelings after doing rotations or after reading.

    What does it mean? Has my eye reached its limit? Is there, perhaps, a problem in my brain, the part that is devoted to vision?

Since you are a hyperope, you must get your eye used to working at nearer and nearer distance. It's a very slow and gradual process, but it's sure and safe.

For example, if today you can read clearly at a 20-inch distance with your left eye (the right one is blindfolded), you must work on shortening this distance with time (reading at shorter and shorter distances).

When you are able to read at about a 4-inch distance, you can wear negative lenses so as to create an overload of fogging, which is suitable to achieve the adaptation.

In short:

1. Take a book.
2. Bring it closer till creating fogging.
3. Blink softly till you have a slight feeling of focusing.
4. Overcome this point of fogging/focusing, which creates an adaptation of your visual system. In your case, if you were once able to focus at the 20-inch distance, and now you read and focus at 12 inches, it means that your visual defect has decreased, since your eye has got used to the imposed visual conditions.

Retinal defocus is an optical stimulus that is artificially driven by lenses so as to ensure the adaptation of focusing.

There are two different kinds of defocus: myopic and hyperopic. For myopic defocus for decreasing myopia (focal image is formed in front of the retina): Use positive lenses! Myopic defocus makes the eye become myopic instantaneously with positive lenses so as to ensure a certain decrease of overaccommodation.

Hyperopic defocus, used for decreasing hyperopia (focal image is formed behind the retina), will use a negative lens. It allows us to increase the accommodation gradually with consequent decreasing of the hyperopia itself.

If you carry out the exercises of ocular stretching and gradually increase defocus, the adaptation and improvements will follow. The periods without improvements exist, and this is normal.

In such periods you must go on doing the exercises (especially increasing/ensuring defocus/fogging and adjusting). When you get to a critical point of imperceptible improvements, your focusing ability will undergo an adaptation, transient at the beginning, but later on, it will become steady.

Scientific studies in animals have proved the effects of retinal defocus on changing your refractive status. The animals, which were subjected to different kinds and levels of defocus, demonstrated the eye's adaptation toward either myopia or hyperopia. When you stop training your eyes with defocus (specific for your refractive error), you will also stop having any improvement. If a hyperope goes on doing the exercises of hyperopic defocus, correctly and continuously, he is even likely to develop the opposite error—myopia. On the other hand, a myope who is trained with myopic defocus theoretically could develop hyperopia unless he stops training at the moment when he reaches the emmetropic state. The rule is to use the state of retinal defocus till you reach the awaited level of adjustment (therefore the improvement).

The eyes, as well as the sight, are influenced by your emotional and mental state. It is a very interesting and important issue, since working on our eyes, we also intervene over the blocks and emotional processes that are at the base of the defect itself. The relation between refractive errors and some kinds of characters is well known: a myope is mostly an introverted person, as if he were closed into his own world of narrow vision, within the limits of ability to focus.

A hyperope, on the contrary, is a person who turns his attention "outside," as if there were a danger to avoid—his sight and his inner world are directed toward the distance. There are as many kinds of characters as there are people: we could say that the character represents a kind of "imprinting" that reveals itself through the eyes. Psychotherapeutic techniques, like EMDR (Eye Movement Desensitization and Reprocessing) and EMT (Eye Movement Technique) work on ocular movements so as to resolve emotional conditions and trauma that influence the patient. Here, we can see the direct connection between the eyes, brain, and sight.

According to the same neurolinguistic planing, different parts of the eyes have a certain, direct influence on the brain: looking up toward the left stimulates some parts of the brain in a completely different way from when looking down toward the right. It's interesting that by working on our sight we can influence and modify our own capability of inner perception as well as dealing with the surrounding world.

Different levels of refraction can make us able to either move away from the surrounding world (though fogging) or to embrace it with our sight—and also with our emotions. Body, mind, and soul are the mirrors that reflect our own light into one single mix—which represents the person with all his characteristics. So, we can state that the techniques of working on the eyes have a very strong component for transforming the person. The eyes are the filters for our surrounding world: change them and your perception will be changed, as well as your being and capability of dealing with others.

32. *I wear correcting lenses (undercorrection) and my sight is blurred when I view distances! What do you advise me to do?*

The fact that you are in a perpetual state of overaccommodation (wearing lenses with full correction and viewing near, as it happens almost always indoors, leads you to your viewing *over* 20/20). This condition ruins and makes the natural focusing become lazy. The fact that you are not able to see perfectly in distance is the first step of visual reeducation; the goal is to stimulate the natural capabilities of your eyes—but not of the lenses.

PVS foresees, in its second phase—retinal defocus (to increase visual acuity)—making the eyes become transiently myopic, so as to stimulate an adaptation of visual system (it may happen with or without training lenses).

It is important thing to follow the techniques the right way.

33. *I'm going to put some questions to you about carrying out the techniques, so as to be able to start practicing.*

 a. *Concerning the exercise of stretching "rotations fixing at a point," am I supposed to turn my head on a horizontal level, fixing at a point (as if I were shaking my head, No), or should I carry out an imaginary circle with my head, fixing a point?*

 b. *Which exercise is the most important, "rotations fixing at a point" or "cyclorotations"?*

 c. *In the Basic Level Program, are you talking about rotations with open eyes (stretching variant for rotations fixing at a point) fixing at a point at over 10 feet of distance, or about those that are described as a "stretching variant for cyclorotations," as if we wanted to follow the borders of a very big clock? If the latter is the right one, how could I fix at a point if I'm carrying out rotations with my eyes?*

 d. *As for stretching in the static position, but not the circular one: For how long am I supposed to keep a certain position? Maybe I shouldn't stay still in one position but alternate with certain rhythm and speed?*

 e. *As for taking breaks while working on reading with positive training lenses: For how long am I supposed to read before having a break? For how long should each break last? Am I supposed to take off the training glasses during these breaks?*

 f. *Is the size of the letters in the text very important when we train to read with training lenses? Which size is the best one?*

g. *Is it true that some people are able to reach visual acuity over 20/20 with the methods of visual reeducation?*

h. *As for different acuity between two eyes: Which difference (in diopters, if possible) requires training with reading with suitable lenses on, blindfolding the weak eye at first, so as to make it equal to the good one? When isn't such a difference important?*

i. *If I understood well, in training with training lenses, the true reading of the text starts after focusing it perfectly with CRB movements, and only at that point should we read it, as long as it's perfectly clear; when the text starts becoming blurred again I must repeat CRB movements and then start reading it again. Or, if after CRB movements the text is still slightly blurred am I supposed to read it?*

j. *Here's a paper with the image of three lines of the text that I gradually made blurred. Can you tell me which one among these lines is to be considered an initial level of fogging of the text to be followed with CRB movements?*

① **To be, or not to be: that is the question**

② **To be, or not to be: that is the question**

③ **To be, or not to be: that is the question**

Here are my answers:

a. The exercise of ocular stretching "rotations fixing at a point" must be carried out so as to let all the extraocular muscles be subjected to the same level of stretching out. If you carried out this exercise only on a horizontal level (as if you were shaking your head, *No*), you would work only on symmetry and coordination of your "right and left" musculus rectus, but not the "superior and inferior" ones, as would happen even nodding *Yes* with your head. "Diagonal" positions must be taken into account.

b. The importance is to be attributed to the level of efficiency. The exercise of "rotations fixing at a point" is more efficient than simple rotations because we directly act over symmetry and coordination between both eyes. Probably, it's very hard to keep "fusion" between the eyes in some extreme parts of the visual field: such a condition shows an imbalance between strength and flexibility of the two eyes. The consequence of such imbalance is a low binocular fixation on one side, and on the other, the lower level of "central fixation" or "centralization." Any shifting from the central fovea leads to a lower quality image. This is the reason why ocular stretching is particularly beneficial for restoring your visual acuity.

c. You can fix at a point, carrying out the rotations with your eyes and keep on fixing at a point at the same time.

d. In the positions of stretching, the time of keeping each single static position itself determines the level of intensity of the exercise: the more you maintain one position, the more intense the exercise will be and, consequently, the level of muscular contraction (agonist) as well as the level of stretching out and lengthening the muscle that is antagonist to the movement. The duration of fixing is approximate and it must be adapted to the initial strength and flexibility of the ocular muscles. The duration must be adapted and lengthened little by little, until the muscle gets used to the load, or the intensity (the relationship of ocular range/duration of contraction). Like in the exercise of retinal defocus, if you don't increase the training stimulus gradually, the adaptation and consequently the improvement in visual acuity would stop.

e. The duration of the breaks is approximate and must be adapted to each person, so trust your feelings. As soon as you feel ready, go on doing the exercises of retinal defocus. I advise you to take the training glasses off during the breaks.

f. There's no perfect size: the basic factor is to create slight fogging, to make the text become slightly blurred, trying to focus the letters.

g. What is usually called "emmetropia" is a simple convention: such convention is still at 20/20 visual acuity, according to the Snellen table. Monkeys, and generally all wild animals, have more or less clear levels of "hyperopia," as it would be defined concerning this "convention." We could develop the visual acuity over 20/20 with PVS. If man had stayed wild, without being constantly exposed to the state of overaccommodation due to narrow places (indoors), probably 21/20 or even more would have been considered as normal visual acuity. The way to run so as to overcome 20/20 is the same one that the myope must run to recover from his refractive error. The exercises are the same: muscular training and retinal defocus. The only difference is that a myope works with low positive lenses (for example, +1), but the person who wants to overcome 20/20 must ensure a suitable state of retinal defocus with +8 diopters. It's important to increase visual-acuity viewing in distance and maintain it in viewing near; otherwise we run the risk of developing hyperopia (farsightedness with little adjustment at near distance). It's up to every single person to see when is the right moment to finish working with defocus.

h. We shouldn't care a lot when the difference in adjusting/ focusing between two eyes (anisometry) is 0.25. If it is higher, at first, we should work on the weaker eye (which suffers from a greater visual defect) to take it to the same level as the other one. You can work on both of your eyes at the same time.

i. You have understood everything completely well: the work you carry out must be with slight fogging (moving the text away or bringing it nearer; it depends whether it's a matter of myopia or hyperopia), the CRB movements, focusing. Then repeat the sequence.

j. The higher the level of fogging with which you are able to focus well, the higher the level of adaptation and consequently the improvement for your eyes. For fogging as in number 3 in your image, adjust with CRB movements until the image is more in focus, like number 1. Then, repeat the sequence, if possible, moving the text away.

34. *Before starting to do the exercises, I have a few questions. Am I supposed to start training with focusing after having trained my ocular muscles for some time (days? weeks? months?) or should I start doing both at the same time? I wear correcting glasses for myopes with 4.5 D lens on my right eye and 4.0 D on the left one. In a training session without my glasses (I hold a book at about a 12-inch distance), only my less myopic eye (the left one) works. Should I train with focusing, putting additional positive lenses over my correcting glasses so as to make both my eyes work, or should I train without my glasses, blindfolding my right eye till it reaches the same level of myopia as my left eye?*

Every myopic person has stiff and inflexible extrinsic ocular muscles, due either to misusing or not using them. Misuse means both abuse in wearing glasses (for example, at near distance where adjustment is possible even without lenses) and wearing glasses when you don't really need them at all, in "safe" places—at your home.

"Preliminary" work—before starting training with retinal defocus —with or without lenses is needed, because those stiff and poorly flexible muscles penalize all your work with retinal defocus, jeopardizing your improvements. Purely "muscular" preliminary work (the active stretching as described in PVS) allows you to have better results in training with retinal defocus since the muscles become more able to relax and focus.

Another great advantage of the preliminary work is the result of restoring the right ocular muscles' symmetry: correcting "wrong" positions that over time will lead to adaptations of the ocular muscles, which may even lose their symmetry (equal relationship between strength/flexibility of all six ocular muscles).

The quality of adjustment depends additionally on the capability of central fixation/centralization (the capability of adjusting or "pointing" the image on the central fovea). This work is aimed at restoring the capability of centralization/central fixation and better muscular symmetry. This can give only "visible" advantages, above all when focusing in the presence of retinal defocus (carrying out the second phase of the PVS program).

Even though the retinal defocus technique isn't widespread, it would be wrong to state that it doesn't exist or that it is inefficient. Your eyes will show it to you after you have carried out the specific training with retinal defocus for some time.

When should you start working with retinal defocus? The very same rule of common sense works here: always follow the principle of retinal defocus.

There's no standard time before starting to train with defocus. However, you should start with the first phase of PVS, carrying out active stretching with your oculomotor muscles and making them work at a maximum range of the visual field.

I advise you to work, at first, with retinal defocus on your "weaker" eye. You can do it by blindfolding your "better" eye and training with retinal defocus on the other eye until both eyes are at an equal refractive level. At that time you can start working with retinal defocus with both eyes.

35. *I work as a dental technician and I would like to know whether my job environment may jeopardize my sight recovery, doing the exercises.*

The answer is *Yes.* One's job environment as well as the life one leads acts on our refractive state, since we get used to our visual environment. Constant near-work can make focusing at a near distance (the process of accommodation) "become chronic," staying in such a state even when accommodation isn't needed—as when viewing in distance (at infinite distance).

Such near-work conditions, over time, may lead to a "spasm of accommodation," where the ciliary muscle is in a state of chronic contraction, thus creating pseudomyopia or transient myopia. Over time it usually gets worse and steady (it becomes an axial lengthening of the ocular globe). This result has its equivalent physiological explanation and is one of the ascertained causes for myopia development: a prolonged state of hyperopic defocus.

According to the theory of defocus, the retina is subjected to repeated adaptations, depending on the position of focus. This simply means that the eye acts as a camera with an autofocusing system, constantly varying focus according to the distance of the observed object and therefore the position of focus—the position of the image on the retina.

According to the theory of retinal defocus, the condition of constantly maintaining the focus *behind* the retina, over time, creates axial myopia, with the consequent lengthening of the ocular globe. This is the characteristic result of medium and high myopia. Such axial lengthening is the result of retinal adaptation (and eye length) to one excessively confined—in time and proximity—to that "near" environment.

Accepting this theory as the accurate one, the opposite can work as well: if the focus is maintained *in front of* the retina (creating myopic defocus instead of the hyperopic one), the retina will constantly be trying to modify the focal level to the focal point, consequently stimulating the relaxation of accommodation that leads to better visual acuity and decreased myopia.

One of the principles of visual reeducation in the Power Vision System is based on this theory: using suitable retinal defocus we can lead the eye to adapt its refractive ability and decrease the initial refractive error until, possibly, compensating for the error. Such results have been obtained in experiments in many animals that were subjected to different states of retinal defocus.

Coming back to your question: one's refractive ability directly depends on the quantity and the kind of optical stimuli she's subjected to, either at near or in distance. According to the theory of accommodative balance, if the near-distance stimuli prevail, they may lead to myopia development.

There are two solutions for this problem:

1. Lessen (or eliminate) near-distance stimuli (changing the type of work with one that allows you to space your sight). This obviously isn't an acceptable solution.

2. Don't let your eyes be subjected to overaccommodative stress, even though you are carrying out near-work. You can obtain the latter result simply by wearing positive lenses whenever carrying out near-work. The process of accommodation has positive effects on focusing at near distance, allowing better focusing ability and visual acuity. Wearing positive lenses in near-distance activities, you can prevent your eyes from excessive near stimuli. This is a great protection against developing myopia.

The dioptric power of the lenses is to be calculated according to one's refractive error and personal needs. An oculist or an optometrist should prescribe the right lens dioptric power.

36. *I'm a myope, –6 and –7 D and 1.25 astigmatism per each eye. Shouldn't I let the muscles that are responsible for adjustment go? I feel as if I have blocked them. I think that using body-building methods, which worked well in your case, wouldn't be useful for me. Perhaps they could even be dangerous. My eyes see as they like and they can't be manipulated like biceps muscles.*

    When training to visualize an object, I'm not able to keep it still and fixed in my mind: it goes away, escapes, runs around my mind, and doesn't let itself be observed in all its details. The same thing happens with my myopia. Whatever I do, it's as if it were completely useless, as if it were to pay for my impatient ego, which has always been looking to cancel my unconscious part and all the processes in my body. Please, in your opinion, how could I improve my visualization, speaking in psychological terms? What do you think about my relationship with my mental images and how could I, gently, lead them to fixation?

You do not need to understand the psychological bases of your myopia, nor the reasons for your impatient ego, to be able improve your ability of focusing. In your case, just being willing to understand could be a symbol and the proof of a much too analytic personality—"brain type"—that is characteristic of myopic people who tend to "make a concept" of everything. Despite very strong psychological components that are hidden behind every visual and bodily process (as proved in psychosomatic medicine), it isn't the most important thing. You don't need to psychoanalyze yourself to resolve or lessen your problem.

You don't have to analyze the image in front of your eyes so as to see it; the only thing you have to do is to simply let the image pass through your eyes. You must work on visual rehabilitation very hard, train and do the exercises, without having psychotherapy.

A normal capability of focusing requests "dynamic relaxation" of the extrinsic ocular muscles, and (as you say) "you should let them go." But how to do it and how to let them relax from chronic tension, which blocks their natural capability of "saccadic vibrating" and "central fixation/centralization"?

A famous school proposes more or less specific exercises of "relaxation." From my long, personal experience and in my opinion, simple muscular relaxation isn't enough to alleviate completely the chronic muscular tension of an overcontracted muscle. It is necessary to restore the physiological muscular qualities like strength and flexibility.

In such a sense, you can train doing the exercises of pure muscular work like active static stretching: simple, but *very* efficacious exercises for decreasing muscular tension and for better centralization.

In this first phase of pure muscular work (you don't have to go to the gym to do the exercises), you must work with suitable retinal defocus, with or without lenses on (*suitable* means that the level of defocus must be calculated on the basis of your own refractive error).

Little by little, as long as your sight is being improved (if you do the exercises constantly and with perseverance), all that's psychological and beyond your myopia will be gradually restored. Then you will probably see that your capability of visualizing is getting better, as well as your memory, and (as it happened to me) also your dealing with people. Additionally, you will trust in life and in the power of self-healing much more.

37. *I'm almost thirty-two and I've been living with myopia ever since I was fourteen. The problem is that I've grown up, but my refractive error is still increasing, very slowly. In all these years everybody has thought that my myopia is a genetic condition and can't be stopped. (I've seen many ophthalmologists and university professors, read books on ophthalmology, and I hope I'll take my degree in medicine very soon.) At this point, I can't do anything else but hope that all these ophthalmologists could be denied.*

It's true (as you know it well, since you study medicine) that it's very hard to overcome the theories and scientific dogmas in any field—especially in the medical one. Who would dare to question an already accepted theory? Now, too many previous certainties are questioned and the standard mantra about genetics is wearing thin. With time, then, the box-camera theory will collapse because of all the evidence against it. This book is about results that people can have by daring to overcome such obsolete paradigms. This means healing and recovering their distance vision to normal by clearing their refractive errors. Science must always evolve but never become blind and imprison itself, unless it wants to run the risk of becoming obsolete by its own dogmas. True science should always question methods that have been handed down to us by a traditional quick-fix philosophy. Nowadays society is more interested in putting on correcting glasses than in allowing people to know the truth about their eyes.

The answer, of course, is up to you—after reading the book. You'll carefully study the PVS physiological bases, and above all else (you should be constant in doing the exercises), you'll have a chance to see the results with your own eyes.

I hope you'll take a specialization in ophthalmology: probably you'll become a pioneer in the field, having read and learned all that is written about the Power Vision System.

39. *I've identified three people who seem to be interested and motivated to carry out the Power Vision visual rehabilitation program. All three cases have the following training schedule: Ocular stretching three days per week, three times per day, wearing positive +2.50 lenses on each eye in all activities that allow it (reading, working at computer).*

   a. Marco (my son): –6.25 right eye (RE) –5.50 left eye (LE) (asymmetry due to cheratoconus). After having trained for four weeks, now he usually wears –5.50 RE and –4.75 LE and according to Snellen tables he has full sight now, even though after working (viewing within 10 feet distance) he notices some worsening. He is the only one who doesn't do any exercise regarding fogging/retinal defocus.

   b. Francesca: –1.25 RE and –0.75 LE. Next Sunday she'll finish her first week of training. Her schedule includes also the exercises of defocus/focusing.

   c. Massimo –2.00 per each eye. Same story as Francesca's.

   My questions:

   a. Does the method change depending on age?

   b. Should I correct the training schedules of my three samples?

   c. When is the right time to change the additional lenses? Should they stay the same? Should both myopes and hyperopes always wear the additional lenses in near viewing (a kind of everlasting visual hygiene)?

   d. Marco has told me that he feels better (and sees better) wearing his present glasses. When is the right time to change graduation for distant viewing?

Entire ocular capabilities must be used so as to maintain ocular strength, flexibility, and coordination correctly. It can't happen if the sight and its capabilities are imprisoned within a limited visual field, as happens when we view through the framework of our glasses.

Regarding the use of positive +2.5 D lenses, I must warn you that the defocus state is to be modulated and changed masterfully, depending on each type of refractive error and, above all, depending on the entity of the error itself. A –0.50 myope can use and wear positive +1.00 or +2.00 lenses when he carries out near-distant activities (so as to oppose the level of overaccommodation that has come from viewing too-near targets). In the case of higher myopia (for example, 2 D), the accommodative state should be limited by taking off the glasses (if it's a case of medium myopia); it's also useful to decrease the lens dioptric power for distance viewing (negative lenses). A myope like Marco (rather high myopia) should wear undercorrection in near viewing (decrease the lens power for some diopters), or, at least, he could carry out his near-distance activities wearing his present lenses and wearing the positive additional ones (for example, a pair of –6.00 D glasses and another pair of +2.00) over the first ones. In this way he decreases the accommodation and dioptric power at –4.00 D.

The use of retinal defocus and therefore the level of the imposed defocus must be changed depending on aim: low positive lenses are to be worn so as to prevent myopia (to decrease an over-accommodative state), but for decreasing myopia gradually you must work with a higher defocus level, which couldn't be used in ordinary activities without jeopardizing visual acuity. The defocus stimulus is aimed at stimulating a *compensation* for the error as well as at increasing refractive capability, and that's why it must be temporary and limited to training sessions.

To answer your questions:

a. The results differ not so much depending on someone's age as on the time she's been wearing glasses (for how long a time her focusing has been "frozen" and helped with lenses, causing "disuse" or functional atrophy due to misuse).

b. It's okay to carry out ocular stretching exercises three days per week and three times per day, but you should make your "samples" understand that muscular work at maximum ocular range must become their ordinary viewing. That's why they must acquire the healthy habit of short ocular rotations while relaxing in the morning, like while brushing their teeth.

Keep insisting on the exercises of ocular stretching, fixing at a steady point and at the extreme parts of the visual field. Do your best to make your "samples" carry out the exercises correctly, gradually increasing the rotation width and staying on the parts of the visual field where the work is very hard, due to "blocks" (at those places where muscular strength, flexibility, and coordination are limited).

c. The defocus state must be changed, increasing the dioptric power of positive *training* lenses, when one can read a text or letters holding the text in completely extended arms and wearing training lenses. In such a case it would be impossible to work with defocus unless increasing the training lens dioptric power.

As long as we are chronically subjected to overaccommodative stress (near-point stress) without counterbalancing it with distant viewing, it will be necessary to use positive lenses for the purpose of prevention and maintenance. Even only 1 diopter positive "leisure" lenses can prevent myopia development, when we become emmetropes.

d. The graduation for distance vision is changed depending on one's present refractive capability and needs. Some ophthalmologists and optometrists prescribe low undercorrection. However, the limit depends on the person's needs: if you are a driver or pilot or someone whose work requires perfect sight, you must wear full correction. If not, undercorrection works well, wearing it only when necessary for clear vision. Many people wear their glasses (or even worse, contact lenses) even when they can see clearly without them. Such a situation does nothing but worsen the accommodative balance and allow the state of chronic overaccommodation, leading to ever-higher refractive error.

41. *I'm twenty-three and I gave up wearing my glasses when I was eighteen, looking to improve my sight. At that time, my diopter (I was a myope) was just 1 D per each eye with a low astigmatism in my left eye.*

I'm in a much worse situation today! I can hardly go around without my glasses, though I haven't worn them for over five years. The last time I went to the ophthalmologist, I had –2.25 in my right eye and –1.75 in the left one. It's surely much worse today.

I discovered your method, and ever since then I've realized that my sight is getting worse and worse. The first three years without wearing my glasses I was able to keep my myopia almost shifting whenever I could, and, despite everything, my myopia was low.

Now I go to the university and follow your advice. I always study holding the text as far as I can, even though I must read more slowly; I do ocular stretching in front of mirror every second day, and I do my best to view distant whenever I can. I never put my glasses on, only my contact lenses (undercorrection), and only when I play football (three or four times a week).

The day after doing stretching exercises, I see less, my eyes are stiff. And when I do stretching I'm not able to notice any block or knot. I'm doing it as best as I can.

I gave up doing the exercises of defocus with positive lenses +1.00 because my sight wasn't clear the day after doing them. Last year, as soon as I took off my +1.00 glasses I had some clear "pulling," but not anymore. Now I only do defocus without positive lenses, but the result is that my eyes are even more stiff.

I have the feeling that whatever I see is a bit blurred, and my eyes are as hard as crystal. Doing stretching exercises, this feeling gets even greater.

Could this theory of mine be true, that my eyes are getting used to sighting everything and are always blurred? Defocus stimulus doesn't do anything but make me get used to the blur even more.

Since I'm a student I study a lot, even if at the furthest possible distance. Could you suggest an optimal program, perhaps one exercise, even if it is difficult and takes a long time to do? (I can find an hour or two a day.)

Figure Q.1 shows the relationship between recovery time and muscular performance quality increase—in this case muscular strength increase. After being trained, a muscle suffers from physiological performance drop, and later on, with time, it overcomes its initial performance limits (strength increase).

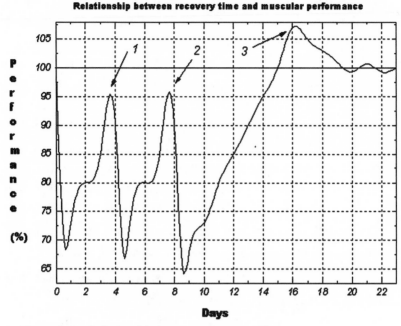

Figure Q.1   *Relationship between Recovery Time and Muscular Performance*

If recovery time is short (as in your case; see also points 1 and 2 in Figure Q.1), the muscle has no time to "overcompensate" and become adapted or increase its strength (overcome the horizontal level of its initial performance).

If recovery time is long enough, you can obtain the necessary adaptation (point 3 in Figure Q.1 in the case of ocular muscles). If recovery time between training sessions of ocular stretching isn't long enough, the result will be a transient and physiological worsening of saccadic vibration and focusing.

If I were you, I would recover much longer, doing the exercises of ocular stretching with two days recovery time at least. The recovery factor is a very personal one and it depends on one's physiological qualities. The training rules regarding ocular muscles are not different from those for any other bodily muscle: both kind of muscles are the striated type and therefore can be trained voluntarily.

So, train but don't forget that any increase in muscular capabilities (even focusing) also depends on the right recovery time and not only on factor of training itself.

42. *I often take a bicycle and ride away, go to the seaside or river to view, observe, and discover what I really see . . . what I'm able to see with my own eyes. In my opinion my sight is a dynamic phenomenon and there's nothing static in it. I have some flashes of clear vision, and the distance at which I'm still able to see clearly is changing every moment. The indoors isn't good for restoring my myopia . . . even though I believe it's not the only reason.*

One's refractive capabilities depend on many different factors like physiological, mental, emotional, or environmental ones.

Having understood all the eye's capabilities of getting used to the induced stimuli—both the near and the distant ones—you can intervene over ocular focusing capability effectively and voluntarily. The refractive state depends on the balance between near and distant stimuli.

The awareness that focusing power is a dynamic phenomenon is the first step toward healing. No human organ nor bodily system makes an exception: when an organ (heart, lungs) undergoes the right stimuli it is pushed toward adaptation. Why should the eyes or refractive system/focusing be an exception?

Do the exercises of ocular stretching and retinal defocus and let me know about your improvements!

43. *I've been doing the exercises from your Power Vision System for two months, because I have very high myopia. I am able to focus on text perfectly, doing CRB movements, and now I hold it at a 5-inch distance (at first it was 6 inches)! Some days ago I thought*

> *I could carry out CRB movement while viewing the landscape (houses, streets, people), and I was able to make my vision clearer and sharper. Now I'm able to distinguish even distant targets and read license plates and registration numbers, billboards, traffic signs—all that was a dense fog before. Yesterday, doing CRB movements, I was able to see perfectly each single rock on the mountain behind my home.*
>
> *Is all this dangerous for my eyes? Can I go on or I should restrict myself to only train by reading a text?*

I'm very glad that you've put the PVS program into practice. Since you've noticed the first improvements and as your refractive capability changes, depending on the specific imposed stimuli, the next step is to keep doing the exercises. It's very important to adapt the training load on the base of already obtained improvement. *Load,* in this case, means the capability of focusing the low state of blur/fogging at ever further distance (for myopia).

Load also means the relationship between the lens power and the reading distance. There's no contraindication for carrying out CRB movements even for distant targets (license plates, billboards), but it is a procedure aimed at restoring the right ocular relaxation, which is necessary for correct focusing. When all the steps of your improvements become stable, you won't need to carry out such a procedure, and you'll be able to see without any effort or will. It's true that CRB movements let you learn how to focus distant targets voluntarily, but the final goal is to make the sight be what it really is: a natural and spontaneous ocular capability.

44. *A year ago I underwent PRK surgery in both eyes as to correct 7 D myopia and astigmatism. Now, a year later, I'm still a myope—*

about 1 D on my right eye (which has always seen less than the dominant left one). After the analysis (corneal topography, and so on), we understood that my myopia is the accommodative type.

With my surgeon's approval, about three months ago, I started training five days a week, with positive lenses only on my right eye (+1, +1.25, +1.50). In the beginning I hardly read 3/10 on Snellen tables. Now, though it isn't easy, I get 9/10. In spite of these very good results, my right eye vision is still unclear. Am I doing everything correctly?

I think that your results speak for themselves. 6/10 improvement in three months is a more than great result, even if your last improvement isn't stable yet.

Passing from +1 to +1.25 and then to +1.50, you've respected load/stimulus increase, the gradual retinal defocus increasing with lenses through the CRB system. You've got the response of your refractive capability and consequently better focusing.

I think you were very lucky because after laser surgery your myopia is still the "accommodative" type. In the opposite case (if your cornea were deformed), the Power Vision System wouldn't help you at all since it acts over extrinsic ocular muscles, the state of tonic accommodation of the ciliary muscle, and the level of central fixation, but not over corneal geometry and its curving.

If the surface of a camera lens is damaged, it is useless to work on the focusing system; it's necessary to repair the lens itself. Since your lens, your cornea after corneal topography, is still good, you can obviously intervene over the focusing system directly, as any other person would.

Keep going this way, which has brought you a 6/10 improvement in three months, and keep going, giving a constant increase of defocus in the eye that needs it. Keep going this way as long as your focusing capability is being increased (when necessary, pass to +2, +2.25).

Any adaptation always follows a gradual stimulation. Listen to your ophthalmologist's advice. She knows everything about your case and can make the right medical diagnosis.

45. *I wear +1.25 lenses at the office (I should correct 1 D) for two hours a day, all week long. Is it reasonable to wear +1 glasses at home, even without reading, and for how long should I do it?*

As long as the eyes are subjected to near-point stress, it's reasonable to do our best to mitigate overaccommodative stress, wearing low undercorrection, or, if necessary, positive lenses (for myopia).

All the activities that require near vision (like reading, writing, working at a computer, or any other kind of indoor work) contribute to such stress. The use of positive "leisure" lenses (in the case of myopia) should be limited to two cases:

a. To prevent myopia that hasn't shown up yet. In this way we can (optically) shift the focal point with lenses, eliminating or mitigating overaccommodative stress (near-point stress).

b. Leisure lenses for stable myopia. We can use them together with (but they cannot replace) ocular stretching or retinal defocus.

As far as I know there's no contraindication for wearing low positive lenses (for low myopia) and low undercorrection for high myopia, indoors and at any other "safe" place (like home). However, when using lenses, a person must consider his own and others' personal safety as well as any possible danger that could come out of slightly blurred vision.

46. *I'm a researcher and I work in Italy, but I also collaborate with some American and Australian universities. Our research deals with experimenting with new treatments for ocular disease and refractive errors. I've been working in a team for over ten years* *and we've been holding congresses worldwide for over thirty years. Every day hundreds of scientists, who know outer and inner ocular structure better than their own pockets, are discovering new techniques that could contribute toward healing ocular pathologies and visual errors.*

We have explored your site very carefully and, at least in the beginning, we were very interested in it, but later on our interest changed into amusement. With time even amusement faded away and was replaced with moral worry.

Only scientists (as we are) can understand that the false promises of "your technique" are aimed only at selling your "magic" book. I would like to let you know that thousands of desperate people would follow anywhere a prophet who preaches curative formulas (which are indecent from a scientific point of view) to resolve their problems.

First, thank you for your e-mail. I'm very sorry I caused amusement among you—the people who work in the ophthalmologic sector—and furthermore, I'm sorry I was your "moral worry."

All that I learned, I did because of the great (unfortunately) ignorance that reigns over refractive errors. Let me add something else: if a "moral worry" must exist, I would look for it in the million-dollar business in glasses, contact lenses, and refractive surgery.

I would like you and your team to give me more solid criticism on what I wrote on my site. I think you should see what I state in my book. I'll personally send you a copy.

I accept any criticism, as long as it's based on scientific facts and reasoning, but not simply saying "You can't."

Only ophthalmology is considered a "closed science": we have been working with the same assumptions for over a hundred years. The first of them is that ocular structure is "fixed," like a camera's, and that it doesn't change depending on someone's visual environment.

One theory on axial myopia (a deformation of the ocular globe) shows that with time, such a deformation (the retina itself) shifts, looking for the right focal point.

I'm sorry that you and your staff see me as a kind of "enemy." It would be much better to weigh thoroughly all that I wrote and experimented on my own eyes, reading my book carefully, examining what I state, and comparing it to scientific deductions. Each of my statements is backed up (as much as I could do so) with scientific works of international value. They are listed in the References.

Changing one's accommodative balance, the average of visual stimuli one gets every day (manipulating his visual environment optically), we can also change his refractive state: at first temporarily, and then summing up all the little adaptations, we can get more stable variations. This happens to myopes when doing the exercises of "disaccommodation" with positive lenses and under-corrected glasses, artificially creating a myopic defocus.

I would like you and your staff not to see me as "a visionary without morals" but as someone who is keen on sight and has spent thousands of hours of his own time studying scientific works. Moreover, I undertook this with my own money, without scholarships or being sponsored by companies that take part in selling or the "business of sight" (as often happens with "worldwide congresses" that are sponsored by such companies). Now, let me ask you something: How much independent judgment is granted to the real and scientific possibility of preventing and of curing myopia, if such congresses are based on and sponsored by "technical sponsors" that are interested in selling, and therefore are not interested in anything that releases consumers from buying glasses, contact lenses, or refractive surgery?

If I threw dust in the blind's eyes I would deserve to become blind myself. On the other hand, if I kept silent on all that I've learned, I would be a partner and ally in a vision business like the current one.

I'm at your complete disposal for any further explanation you need.

48. *I have several questions for you.*

    a. *Myopia is due to excessive ocular bulb elongation. Therefore, it means that one who improves his sight should have ocular bulb shortening. Has anyone checked it out?*

    b. *I have another question for you: Is there any limit concerning the level of myopia that could be cured (perhaps due to the highest level of ocular bulb elasticity that can't be overcome)? Let me explain it better: myopes who practice the exercises reach some improvements that are limited to 1–2 diopters. Does it mean that it is impossible to heal myopia completely if it is higher than these values?*

    c. *When I carry out rotation with my head, I have double vision in two points. There's no binocular focusing. . . . What should I do?*

    d. *Should the ocular relaxation in CRB be simultaneous with blinking, or just follow it?*

    e. *For rotations at extreme points: does it mean that fixing at a steady point at 10-feet distance, the head must rotate while bending downward and then upward, very slowly carry out such movements over and over again, and maintain binocular vision? But . . . my nose hinders binocular vision in lateral zones. So, what should I do?*

    f. *Do you have the phone number of any ophthalmologist or ocular therapist who approves and uses ocular gymnastics?*

Let me answer your questions:

a. Ocular bulb elongating (axial myopia) happens after long-lasting retinal defocus (near-point stress, overuse of lenses and glasses, excessive nervous stress, bad nutrition, and so on). Only *after some time,* transient myopia or pseudomyopia becomes an axial deformation of the ocular bulb. The very same thing works also in the opposite way: it takes *time,* and after some time all the improvements (due to practicing) can improve the ocular bulb form (better focusing, ocular movements, less ocular tiredness). We are in an experimental field (even though the causes of elongation are acknowledged by science as well as tested). My advice is, *Practice* the exercises without conjecturing too much—you don't need it for good results. The will to learn is an advantage, but on the other side, if you stop and conjecture, then it is a disadvantage. What is really important in the Power Vision System is *practicing,* after arranging the exercises depending on your needs (refractive errors, muscular imbalance, retinal defocus entity, the choice of correcting lenses [full correction or undercorrection]).

b. The highest myopia to be cured doesn't exist, nor does the highest theoretical level of myopia development, except the limit of retinal breaking due to excessive axial elongation of the ocular bulb (the latter is another reason to *start* doing something more for your eyes and your myopia besides the *palliatives* of wearing glasses, contact lenses, and refractive surgery). As for the latter point, refractive surgery itself: After undergoing refractive surgery, *no* eye is healthy, despite its ability to focus, because the ocular bulb deformation persists. Furthermore, such deformation can worsen into retinal detachment, with time, and if "myopizating" conditions come back.

Either refractive surgery or the Power Vision System *takes a long time* to see complete improvement. Out of 500 people who learn about PVS, 200 of them practice only during the first month, and only 100 carry out the whole program with *perseverance* till the first results, and only about 50 of them get further results, which come with time. Not all of the latter group are willing and able to link up to the Internet to share their results with others. Unfortunately, we don't have follow-up studies to monitor all the patients throughout time; therefore, at the moment, the results are anecdotal, but not unreliable. With time, as the technique spreads out, more and more voices will be supporting PVS visual rehabilitation. In the meantime, this technique's "pioneers" can be the first to overcome the limits of *myopia* that are imposed by present medical science (and not by scientific experimentation, which has been affirming the refractive state dynamism and changeability *for a long time*). These "pioneers" will experience *benefits* from such preventive methods and treatment.

c. If you don't have fixation and "pointing" in the extreme points of one part of your visual field it means that your agonist and antagonistic ocular muscles suffer from lack of strength and flexibility. Such a condition affects "central fixation/ centralization," or better focusing on the retinal part called the "fovea centralis," which results in blurred vision. Impatience is a bad ally when the journey is very long and requires perseverance and patience.

d. Blinking and relaxation are two synonyms: since you have asked me this question it means that you didn't understand the purpose of blinking—that is, ocular *relaxation* itself.

e. Keep on binocular fixation as long as you can: your nose is a physiological obstacle that must be "taken into account and respected": it doesn't mean that the exercise is less efficacious.

f. The therapists will come with time: ophthalmologists and opticians will become aware of this treatment's importance, little by little. I'm at their complete disposal, whenever they need me. The patient himself must be the one to *ask for nonpalliative* treatment. The patient will ask for "unconventional" methods, as such methods are considered today, and they will substitute for or, at least, add to the present conventional "treatments."

I hope I've satisfied your curiosity. My advice is always the same: *Practice, practice, practice!*

An Interview with David De Angelis

What prompted you to write this book?

I wanted to share my successful experience about the scientific and real possibility of lessening and even completely recovering from refractive errors. I would like, somehow, to awaken people and not only show them a way to heal their refractive errors but also to help them understand that a great many things written by academic authorities aren't the absolute truth. Conventional glasses are not what the authorities want us to believe (a way to heal our sight) but just a palliative remedy, which does nothing else but worsen the initial refractive error.

What do you expect from your readers?

I expect everyone who has eyes for seeing to see and all those who have the ears for hearing to listen. Whoever has the sense to do it now has a new way of healing besides the famous Bates Method. Apart from the price of the book, using this method costs nothing in monetary terms. It is true that a considerable degree of personal commitment and effort is required to do the specific exercises.

Do you think that researchers in ophthalmology or the ophthalmologists themselves could react?

There is no doubt that I will not be appreciated by all those who are stuck to the old and obsolete theories on the human eye's functioning. The human eye is often compared to a camera with fixed focusing, but it isn't so. Eminent authors of scientific studies on this issue and all the results that I've achieved personally prove that it is just a "partial" concept. The eye can change its refractive status, including its focal length. Speaking in technical terms, it means that the length of an eye, and therefore its capability of focus, changes depending on the kind of stimuli it is subjected to on a regular basis (the theory of accommodative balance). Numerous studies of various animal species have proven it: myopic and hyperopic stimuli lead to myopia and hyperopia development in primates (and humans) over time.

These results are due to the proven fact that the retina undergoes specific adaptations and shifting, depending on the position of the focal point of an image. Therefore, the eye isn't a kind of camera with fixed focusing but a very sophisticated camera with autofocusing. Working consciously on the position of focus (through suitable work with gradual retinal defocus), over time, we can get at changing the "default" adjustment. Any organ, according to the SAID (Specific Adaptation to the Imposed Demand) Principle, gets used to any stimulus if it is strong enough and repeated over time. The eyes are not an exception.

What could the professionals (ophthalmologists and the researchers on ophthalmology) be thinking? I've written *The Secret of Perfect Vision* for them too, so as to change their point of view about vision. By understanding the true meaning of the experimental data, the appreciation of the problem can change. This could lead to a broad-based scientific approach that would reduce our dependence on a minus-lens palliative and find a true and better solution by the methods advocated in this book.

The Power Vision System, the masterful use of positive lenses for myopes, may have a great effect in myopia prevention. Myopia is very common nowadays, because of our exposure to constant near-point stress (the theory of accommodative balance).

The author is available to his readers on his website (www.power-visionsystem.com) for further details and explanations about theoretical bases of the system and about using it in practice. He can be reached by e-mail at powervision@powervisionsystem.com. A support forum is available at www.powervisionforum.com.

Before sending an e-mail, please read the FAQ section and do a search in the support forum.

Appendix 1

The Norms of Sight Preservation

The following rules will help prevent you from developing visual disorders and from misusing and abusing your eyes, the greatest mistake many people make. We should remember that little differences in our lifestyles and the way we carry out our ordinary gestures, exercises, behavior, thoughts, and emotions may either improve or worsen our sight and our lives.

1. *Don't abuse the wearing of correcting glasses.* Wear them (in case of low myopia) only when necessary: when required by the law and by safety rules. Don't ever wear them to view at near distance when you can focus well without correcting lenses (for myopes).

2. *Wear undercorrection whenever possible.* Whenever you can (at safe places, at your home, for example), wear undercorrection (1 or 0.50 less than your ordinary dioptric power) or, in case of a very low myopia, get used to not wearing glasses at all.

3. *Don't abuse wearing sunglasses.* Limit wearing sunglasses to when desperately needed because of a too-high daze (for example, on the mountain, on the seaside in summertime).

4. *Don't work or read at too short a distance.* Work or read at the furthest distance at which you're still able to focus well (so as to limit overaccommodative stress).

5. *Avoid taking positions that cause asymmetric development of ocular muscles.* Watching TV lying on the bed, or reading and holding your head inclined (not perpendicular to the line you are reading) leads to extrinsic ocular muscles' asymmetry, with consequent loss in their mobility and coordination as well as central fixation or centralization on the central fovea.

6. *Maintain practice with the Power Vision System.* Even without having sight disorders and after having obtained clear distance sight with this method, continue doing the exercises of ocular stretching.

7. *Enjoy every miraculous day of sight.* Look at sunshine, blue seawater, mountains, and the light in your dear one's eyes with the astonishment and enthusiasm of someone who has spent a great deal of his life imprisoned in the "fog" and "darkness" of an already forgotten myopia.

Training Programs

Basic Level (building basic strength and flexibility)

One day a week:

- Do the exercises of ocular stretching, once with eyes open and once with your eyes closed.
- Do a slow and concentrated rotation with the open eyes, fixing at a point that is at the maximum level of stretching (three times on one side and three times on the opposite one), trying to maintain ocular fusion.
- Do slow and concentrated rotations with your eyes closed (ten times on one side and ten times on the opposite one).

Every day (except Sunday):

- Train for 30 minutes with training glasses on (positive lenses or undercorrected glasses for myopes and negative ones for hyperopes).
- Make your eyes used to bright light (wear sunglasses as infrequently as possible).

Medium Level (medium/fast improvements)

Two days a week:

- Do two sessions a day (at least 4 hours recovery time is needed between two training sessions).
- Do exercises of ocular stretching, twice with your eyes closed and twice with your eyes open.
- Do slow and concentrated rotations with open eyes, fixing at a point that is at the highest level of stretching (five times on one side and five times on the opposite one), trying to maintain ocular fusion.
- Do slow and concentrated rotations with your eyes closed (five times on one side and five times on the opposite one).

Every day (except Sunday):

- Train for an hour with training glasses on (positive lenses or undercorrected glasses for myopes and negative ones for hyperopes).
- Make your eyes used to the bright light (wear sunglasses as infrequently as possible).

Advanced Level (super-fast program, fast results)

This program was developed for those people who are strongly motivated to improve the capability of their accommodation system. This program requires *great* concentration and dedication in doing the exercises, each and every day, with *great* consistency.

On Monday, Wednesday, and Friday or three other alternate days; in the morning, afternoon, and evening (4 hours of recovery time is needed between training sessions):

- Do the exercises of ocular stretching; twice with eyes open and twice with your eyes closed.

- Do slow and concentrated rotations with open eyes, fixing at a point that is at the highest level of stretching (ten times on one side and ten times on the opposite one), trying to maintain ocular fusion.

- Do slow and concentrated rotations with your eyes closed (ten times on one side and ten times on the opposite one).

Every day (except Sunday):

- Train for 2 hours with your training glasses on (positive lenses or undercorrected glasses for myopes and negative ones for hyperopes).
- Make your eyes used to the bright light (wear sunglasses as infrequently as possible).

It is very important to wear correcting lenses as *infrequently* as possible (for example, at home or when having a walk) except in carrying out duties and tasks for which wearing correcting lenses is compulsory by law and for safety reasons. Myopes who suffer from very high myopia—for example, over 4 or 5 diopters—must wear correcting lenses, but they should wear undercorrection whenever possible.

In this phase the eyes are subjected to a specific stress (*specific* meaning the stress we create voluntarily by specific work, which leads to visibly better accommodation and visual disorder lessening). Such visual stress may create a different phenomena: the most usual and the ordinary ones are a light headache and some pain in the ocular muscles. This is completely normal, since any bodily muscle (while being trained) is subjected to stress (therefore the pain) before changing its physiology, strength, and flexibility.

Little by little, by continuing with your training, your ocular muscles will get used to the training load and the pains will gradually disappear, showing a clear sign of muscular adaptation: greater muscular strength and flexibility, as well as the improvement of the functioning of your accommodation system.

Keep in mind: Training protocols in PVS can and must be made suitable for each specific visual defect and its manifestation. The protocols described are just indicative, since presently they are not standardized in a huge sample of people.

Appendix 3

The Origin and History
of Visual Standards

The visual standard in use in the early twentieth century was the sharpest vision that could be obtained by use of a minus lens (20/20). During World War I, this standard was determined to be excessively high and therefore unreasonable; a great many soldiers would be wearing minus glasses if this standard were enforced. It was decided to not use the 20/20 standard and to choose 20/40 as reasonable and acceptable.

If you are working to achieve a standard of vision, I suggest using the 20/40 standard rather than using a strong minus lens to get to 20/20. The exception would be for driving a car at night. This is a reasonable and practical way to meet requirements and not have your natural eyes adapt to the minus lens any more than is necessary.

Keep in mind: The 20/40 standard was done under room illumination. That is the legal requirement. In deep darkness you will get readings of 20/70 or so, but the Department of Motor Vehicles does not test for deep dusk conditions. Strong consistent work with a plus lens can help you clear your "dusk" vision to 20/40 or better—providing you have the motivation to do so. Be wise and be careful.

More information is available at www.myopiafree.com.

How to Make Your Own Snellen Chart

To calculate the height of the letters, use the Radian angle measurement system.

Thus:

5 minutes-of-angle = 0.001455 Radians

Then:

12 – 20 = 240 inches

240 – 0.001455 = 0.35 inches at 20 feet

So we should say 20/20/0.35 inches to be clear.

Obviously you can obtain the 20/40-sized letter by multiplying 0.35 – 2 = 0.70 inches. The same holds for 20/80-sized characters.

Using these calculations, you can set up a chart for 10 feet. You can easily calculate the size of the letters and cut them out of the newspaper.

The Concept of Legal Ownership

Legal Conditions for a Preventive Effort with Engineer-Scientists and Embry-Riddle

In order to conduct a nearsightedness prevention effort, it is necessary to establish the person who has legal ownership and control of your visual future. I was asked to sketch out the legal requirements for a preventive effort at a four-year aeronautical engineering college.

The following would be the basis for a "legal ownership agreement" and responsibility, leading to a signed statement with the Embry-Riddle students who would enter into this type of near-sightedness prevention study. If I were entering a four-year college, and I valued my distance vision, I would have no problem signing a contract of this nature as part of a scientific-engineering study.

My eyes belong to me. I am responsible for my body and my eyes. They are mine. I can delegate some responsibility to a third party but that third party should never assume they own my eyes or have legal control over my eyes.

There is an assumption that I have totally transferred legal control over my eyes to an optometrist by entering his office. But this is only an assumption and is not justified by most ethical standards.

What I expect from a professional in the field of health care is a discussion of alternatives when the alternative is feasible. This must be an active process on the part of the person who will help me and on my part also.

I expect alternatives (even difficult alternatives like prevention with a plus lens) to be discussed, with the issue of effective prevention clearly identified as the second opinion. Since my eyes legally belong to me, it would be up to me to go out and research the true effect that a minus lens has on the refractive status of the natural eye.

If I decided that effective prevention was not in my future, or for any other reason, then I would transfer legal control to the optometrist and accept the long-term effect and consequences of using a minus lens on my eyes constantly.

If all health care professionals broached this type of discussion of your legal ownership of your own eyes, a better working relationship could be developed among pilots, engineers, scientists, and optometrists. Legal responsibility would remain with the individual. There would be no implicit transfer of control at all. The person would be mature enough to understand her responsibility in asserting control over the refractive status of her own eyes.

The concept of legal ownership and personal responsibility is currently broken by the traditional use of the minus lens as a quick fix.

Glossary

Accommodation: Capability of correctly adjusting images at any distance.

Accommotrac Vision Trainer: Patented system of visual reeducation by machine, which sets up a visual/sound biofeedback system, to let you get used to the correct adjustments at different distances.

Active, static stretching: Technique used in the Power Vision System; consists of contracting the agonist muscle and extending/stretching out the antagonistic one (referring to one single portion and one ocular movement). It is aimed at training the eyes at the maximum range of their movement, thus overcoming possible blocks in some parts of visual field (these parts show negative imbalance of muscular mass in the extrinsic ocular muscles).

Biofeedback: Technique that allows you to train so as to become able to control physiological functions that aren't normally subject to voluntary control. It uses visual and/or sound feedback.

Blur-driven accommodation: Physiological response used in the Power Vision System to stimulate adjustment and gradually eliminate refractive error. It's used in opposite ways in myopia and hyperopia.

Central fixation: Capability of a normal/emmetropic eye to make a focused image fall on the central part of central fovea.

Central fovea: The part of the retina where the image must fall so as to have perfect adjustment.

Ciliary muscle: A smooth-type muscle not subject to voluntary control. It is one of the causes of refractive errors.

Circular respiration: Particularly efficacious respiration for maintaining the body in homeostasis and psychosomatic equilibrium. This method is used in Rebirthing, Vivation, and olotropic respiration in order to lead a person into unordinary states of consciousness and further to lead him to a transpersonal sphere.

"Correcting" lenses: Ordinarily prescribed lenses for full (and transient) correction of any visual error.

CRB movement: Specific movement that allows us to stimulate and induce the process of accommodation by muscular work.

Flashes of clear vision: The people who carry out visual reeducation know this phenomenon well: it's characterized by moments when a myopic person is able to see very clearly, much better than usual.

Fogging: *See* Blur-driven accommodation.

Gradual undercorrection: Procedure by which you gradually become used to wearing undercorrected lenses (compared with the normal prescription) so as to maintain the benefits of visual training without creating the negative state of undercorrection.

Homeostasis: Capability of the living body to maintain its stability and inner order, ensuring control of change due to external changes. The word defines a control system in physiological systems.

Hyperopic defocus: If dioptric stimulus is gradually being shifted beyond optical infinity (possible only using optical systems), the accommodative response is gradually being increased, moving away from tonic accommodation.

Laser refractive surgery: Also known as **LASIK;** surgical method for resolving refractive errors. The techniques and methods are constantly being developed, but they are very invasive and act over physiological structures that, once trained, don't maintain their original characteristics of physiological functioning. The two greatest problems are that refractive surgery doesn't act on the real causes of refractive errors (acting in merely a "mechanical" way) nor do they recognize the possibilities of self-modifying and ocular adaptation, which is of course the purpose of visual training. The long-term effects of LASIK are still unknown.

Myopia: The most common refractive error; when viewing distantly, the image of the observed object falls in front of the retina (therefore it's blurred).

Myopic defocus: Occurs when an accommodative stimulus overcomes someone's personal accommodation width for 1–2 diopters, creating greater underaccommodation and consequently an unfocused image. Beyond this point, the accommodative response becomes lower and lower, and gradually moves toward tonic accommodation.

Norms of visual prevention: Particular behaviors that prevent us from developing refractive errors. People who have obtained clear, distinct sight again, through visual training, can maintain it using these norms.

Overaccommodation (or **overaccommodative stress**): The main reason for sight deteriorating, according to the theory that sees the environment and someone's visual habits as the reasons for refractive error development. Caused by either excessive nearwork or wearing "correcting" glasses even at a distance where one normally can focus well and correctly.

Power Vision System: Currently the most efficacious visual training system; characterized by exercises that act over functional refractive disorders directly, but not in an invasive way.

Retinal defocus: A specific stimulus by which the eye is led to changing its refractive state, over time. There are two kinds of retinal defocus: myopic defocus (focus in front of the retina) and hyperopic (focus behind the retina).

SAID Principle: Specific Adaptation to the Imposed Demand; the basic principle for the Power Vision System. According to this principle, the eyes adapt their structure and functioning depending on a specific stimuli.

Strabismus/Squint: Condition where the eyes point in different directions, causing double vision or visual suppression of one eye (not the dominant one).

Training lenses: Used in Power Vision System to strengthen the accommodative stimulus. They are opposite in sign to the ordinarily prescribed ones: positive lenses for myopes and negative lenses for hyperopes.

Visual axis' convergence: Ocular capability of maintaining the exact and symmetric convergence, fixing at near-distant objects and in all the sections of visual field.

Visual training: Techniques aimed at restoring refractive errors naturally in a noninvasive way.

References

Bates, W. H. (1981) The Bates Method for Better Eyesight without Glasses. Owl Books. Originally published 1920.

Beatty, J., & Wagoner, B. L. (1978) Pupillometric signs of brain activation with level of cognitive processing. Science 199, 1216–1218.

Birnbaum, M. H. (1984) Nearpoint visual stress: a physiological model. J. Am. Optom. Assoc. 55, 825–835.

Birnbaum, M. H. (1985) Nearpoint visual stress: clinical implication. J. Am. Optom. Assoc. 56, 480–490.

Birnbaum, M. H. (1988) Myopia and near-point stress model. In Myopia & Nearwork, p. 169. Butterworth Heinemann.

Birnbaum, M. H. (1993) Optmometric Management of Nearpoint Vision Disorders. Butterworth Heinemann.

Cannon, W. B. (1929) Bodily Changes in Pain, Hunger, Fear and Rage. An Account of Recent Researches into the Function of Emotional Excitement. Appleton.

Catania, A. (1964) On the visual acuity of the pigeon. J. Exp. Anal. Behav. 7, 361–366.

Curtin, B. J. (1985) The Myopia. Basic Science and Clinical Management. Harper & Row.

Ehrlinch, D. L. (1987) Near vision stress: vergence adaptation and accommodative fatigue. Ophthal. Physiol. Opt. 7, 353–357.

Fitzke, F. W., Hayes, W., Holden, A. L. (1985) Refractive sectors in the visual field of the pigeon eye. J. Physiol. (Lond.) 369, 33–44.

Gottlieb, R. L. (1982) Neuropsychology of myopia. J. Optom. Vis. Dev. 13, 3–27.

Grosvenor, T., Goss, D. A. (1999) Clinical Management of Myopia. Butterworth Heinemann.

Hayden, R. (1941) Development and prevention of myopia at the United States naval academy. The American Medical Association, Vol. 25 (old series Vol. 82), Nr. 4.

Hess, E. H., Polt, J. M. (1964) Pupil size in relation to mental activity during simple problem-solving. Science 143, 1190–1192.

Holt, W. R., Caruso, J. L., Riley, J. B. (1978) Transcendental Meditation versus pseudo-meditation on visual choice reaction time. Perceptual and Motor Skills, n. 46, p. 726.

Hung, L. F., Crawford, M. L. J., Smith, E. L. (1995) Spectacle lenses alter eye growth and the refractive status of young monkeys. Nature Medicine, n. 1, pp. 761–765.

Irving, E. L., Callender, M. G., Sivak, J. G. (1991) Inducing myopia, hyperopia and astigmatism in chicks. Opt. Vis. Sci., n. 68, pp. 364–368.

Irving, E. L., Sivak, J. G., Callender, M. G. (1992) Refractive plasticity of the developing chick eye. Ophthal. Physiol. Opt. 12, 448–456.

Kahnemann, D. (1973) Attention and Effort pp. 1–49. Prentice-Hall.

Kuhn, T. S. (1996) The Structure of Scientific Revolutions, 3rd ed. University of Chicago Press.

Libby, W. L., Lacey, B. C., Lacey, J. I. (1973) Pupillary and cardiac activity during visual attention. Psychophysiology 10, 270–294.

Lowen, Alexander. (1994) Bioenergetics. Compass Books.

McBrien, N. A., Norton, T. T. (1992) The development of experimental myopia and ocular component dimension in monocularly lid-shrews. (Tupaia belangeri). Vis. Res. 32, 843–852.

McFadden S., Wallman, J. (1995) Guinea pig eye growth compensates for spectacle lenses. Invest. Ophthalmol. Vis. Sci. 36 (ARVO Suppl.), S758.

Medina, A. (1987) A model for emmetropization: the effects of correcting lenses. Acta Ophthalmol. Nr. 65, S. 565–571.

Medina, A., Fariza, E. (1993) Emmetropization as a first-order feedback system. Vis. Res. 33, 21–25.

Miles, F. A., Wallman, J. (1990) Local ocular compensation for imposed local refractive error. Vis. Res. 30, 339–349.

Millodot, M., Blough, P. M. (1971) The refractive state of the pigeon eye. Vis. Res. 11, 1019–1022.

Norton, T. (1990) Experimental myopia in tree shrews. In Myopia and the Control of the Eye Growth. Ciba Foundation Symposium 155 (F. R. Bock and K. Widdows, eds), pp. 178–199. Wiley.

Nye, P. W. (1973) On the functional differences between frontal and lateral visual fields of the pigeons. Vis. Res. 13, 559–574.

Oakley, K. H., Young, F. A. (1975) Bifocal control of myopia. Am. J. Optom. Physiol. Opt. 52, 758–764.

Ong. E., Ciuffreda, K. J. (1995) Nearwork-induced transient myopia: a critical review. Doc. Ophtalmol. 91, 57–85.

Ong, E., Ciuffreda, K. J. (1997) Accommodation, Nearwork and Myopia. Optometric extension Program.

Paliaga, G. P. (1995) I vizi di refrazione. Edizioni Minerva Medica.

Pribram, K., Mcguinness, D. (1975) Arousal, activation and effort in the control of attention. Psychol. Rev. 82, 116–149.

Raviola, E., Wiesel, T. N. (1985) An animal model of myopia. N. Engl. J. Med 312, 1609–1615.

Reynolds, H., M.D. (1941). Development and Prevention of Myopia at the United States Naval Academy Vol. 25 (old series Vol. 82), no. 4.

Roberts, W., Banford, R. (1967) Evaluation of bifocal correction of juvenile myopia. Optom. Weekly 58, 25–31, 21 Sept.; 58, 21–30, 28 Sept.; 58, 23–28, 5 Oct.; 58, 27–34, 12 Oct.; 19–26, 26 Oct.

Robinson, D. A. (1964) The mechanics of human saccadic eye movement. J Physiol. 174, 245–264.

Rosenfield, M., Abraham-Cohen, J. A. (1999) Blur sensitivity in myopes. Optom. Vis. Sci. 76(5), 303–307.

Rosenfield, M., Ciuffreda, K. J., Novogradsky, L. (1992) Contribution of accommodation and disparity-vergence to transient nearwork-induced myopic shifts. Ophthal. Physiol. Opt. 12, 433–436.

Rosenfield, M., Gilmartin, B. (1999) Accommodative error, adaptation and myopia. Ophtalmic Physiol. Opt., 19(2), 159–164.

Schaeffel, F., Glasser, A., Howland, H. C. (1988) Accommodation, refractive error and eye growth in chickens. Vis. Res. 28, 639–657.

Schaeffel, F., Howland, H. C. (1991) Properties of feedback loops controlling eye growth and refractive state in the chicken. Vis. Res. 31, 717–734.

Scott, A. B. (1994) Change of eye muscle sarcomeres according to eye position. J. Ped. Ophtalmol. and Strab., 31(2), 85–88.

Selys, H. (1956) The Stress of Life. McGraw-Hill.

Siegwart, J. T., Norton, T. T. (1993) Refractive and ocular changes in tree shrews raised with plus or minus lenses. Invest. Ophthalmol. Vis. Sci. 34 (ARVO Suppl.), S1208.

Skeffington, A. M. (1974) Optometric Extension Program Continuing Education Courses. Optometric Extension Program Foundation. Originally published 1928.

Smith III, E. L. (1998) Environmentally induced refractive errors in animals. In Myopia & Nearwork, p. 73. Butterworth Heinemann.

Smith III, E. L., Hung, L. F. (1995) Optical diffusion disrupts emmetropization and produces axial myopia in young monkeys. Invest. Ophthalmol. Vis. Sci. 36 (Suppl.), 758.

Smith III, E. L., Hung, L. F., Harwerth, R. S. (1994) Effects of optically induced blur on the refractive status of young monkeys. Vis. Res. 34, 293–301.

Suchoff, I. B., Petito, G. T. (1986) The efficacy of visual therapy: accommodative disorders and nonstrasbismic anomalies of binocular vision. J. Am. Opt. Ass. 17, 119–125.

Trachtman, J. N. (1978) Biofeedback of accommodation to functional myopia: a case report. Am. J. Optom. Physiol. Opt. 55, 400–486.

Trachtman, J. N. (1986) Perceptual correlates of accommodative biofeedback training. Research Reports and Special Articles, Optom Extension Program, 59(3), 1.

Trachtman, J. N., Jambalvo, V., Feldman, J. (1981) Biofeedback of accommodation to reduce functional myopia: a case report. Biofeedback and Self Regulation 6, 546–64.

Wallman, J. (1993) Retinal control of eye growth and refraction. Prog. Retinal Res. 12, 134–153.

Wallman, J., Adams, J. I. (1987) Developmental aspects of experimental myopia in chicks: susceptibility, recovery and relation to emmetropization. Vis. Res. 27, 1139–1163.

Wildsoet, C. F. (1998) Structural correlates of myopia. In Myopia & Nearwork, p. 35. Butterworth Heinemann.

Wildsoet, C. F., Wallman, J. (1997) Is the rate of lens–compensation proportional to the degree of defocus? Invest. Ophthalmol. Vis. Sci. (ARVO Suppl.), S461.

Young, F. A. (1965) Visual refractive errors of wild and laboratory monkeys. EEENT Digest, August.

Young, F. A. (1971) The Development of Myopia. Contacto.

Young F. A. (1982). Primate miopia. Am. J. Optom. Physiol. Opt. Nr. 58, S. 560–566.

Young, F. A., et al. (1969) The transmission of refractive errors within Eskimos families. Am. J. Opt. and Arch. Am. Acad. Opt., 46(9).

Further Reading

Books and Periodicals

AAVV. Bibliography of Near Lenses & Vision Training Research. Optometric Extension Program. 1998.

Abel, Robert. The Eye Care Revolution. Prevent and Reverse Common Vision Problems. Kensington Publishing. 1999.

Baker, Douglas. Esoteric Anatomy. Baker Publications. 1997.

Barnes, Jonathan. Improve Your Eyesight. Souvenir Press. 2000.

Benjamin, Harry. Better Sight without Glasses. HarperCollins. 1992.

Brown, Otis S. How to Avoid Nearsightedness—A Scientific Study of the Eye's Behavior. C & O Research. 1999. www.myopiafree.org.

Deakins, Fred T., Grossman, Mark R. The New Revolution in Eye Care: Your Complete Guide to Improved Eyesight. America 20/20 Corporation. 2000.

De Angelis, David. Power-Flex Stretching—The Secrets of Super Flexibility. www.powerflexsystem.com.

Friedberg, Fred, & McKay, Matthew. Do-It-Yourself Eye Movement Techniques for Emotional Healing. New Harbinger. 2001.

Goodrich, Janet. Natural Vision Improvement. Ten Speed. 1998.

Huxley, A. The Art of Seeing. Creative Arts. 1982.

Kaplan, Robert Michael. The Power behind Your Eyes. Healing Art Press. 1995.

Kaplan, Roberto. Conscious Seeing—Transforming Your Life through Your Eyes. Beyond Words Publishing. 2002.

Leung, Steve H., Bossino, Han A. You Are Wearing the Wrong Glasses. 2003. www.chinamyopia.org.

Liberman, Jacob. Take Off Your Glasses and See: A Mind/Body Approach to Expanding Your Eyesight and Insight. Three Rivers Press. 1995.

Markert, Cristopher. Seeing Well Again *without* Your Glasses. Prentice Hall. 1983.

Quackenbush, Thomas R. Better Eyesight: The Complete Magazines of William H. Bates. North Atlantic Books. 2001.

Quackenbush, Thomas R. Relearning to See: Improve Your Eyesight—Naturally! North Atlantic Books. 2000.

Rehm, Donald S. The Myopia Myth: The Truth about Nearsightedness and How to Prevent It. International Myopia Prevention Association. 1981. www.myopia.org.

Rosembauer, Wolfgang. Better Vision Naturally. Sterling. 1998.

Rosenfield, Mark, & Gilmartin, Bernard. Myopia & Nearwork. Butterworth Heinemann. 1998.

Rottè, Joanna, & Yamamoto, Koji. Vision: A Holistic Guide to Healing the Eyesight. Japan Publications. 1986.

Roy, Marilyn. Eyerobics: How to Improve Your Vision. Peanut Butter Publishing. 1997.

Schneider, Meir. Meir Schneider's Miracle Eyesight Method: The Natural Way to Heal and Improve Your Vision. Audio cassette. 1997.

Severson, Brian. Vision Freedom. 1998.

Shaftesbury, Edmund. Instantaneous Personal Magnetism. Kessinger Publishing. 1926 (III Department of the Magnetic Eye).

Shapiro, Francine. Eye Movement Desensitization and Reprocessing (EMDR). Guilford Press. 2001.

Schmid, Klaus. Myopia Manual: An Impartial Documentation of All the Reasons, Therapies and Recommendations. Pagefreepublishing. 2004. www.myopia-manual.de.

Sussman, Martin. The Program for Better Vision. North Atlantic Books. 1998.

Totton, Nick, & Edmondson, Em. Reichian Growth Work: Melting the Blocks to Life and Love. Prism Press. 1988.

Websites

www.powervisionsystem.com (official website; free newsletter for subscribers)

www.powervisionforum.com (support forum on vision training and the Power Vision System)

www.chinamyopia.org

www.myopia.org

www.myopia-manual.de

www.myopiafree.com

Index

Acknowledgments

Thanks to all authors who helped me to gain a deep understanding of the "myopia problem" and of its subtle causes. Without their scientific studies and works this book would never have been written.

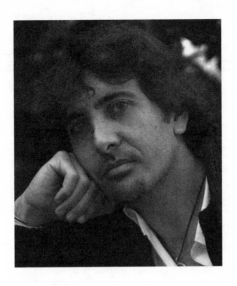

About the Author

David De Angelis received his law degree from La Sapienza University in Rome, but soon became interested in learning more about the body's development and psycho-bodily integration in the wake of muscular rehabilitation techniques and bioenergetics. After a great deal of studying and research, he wrote *Power-Flex Stretching: Super Flexibility and Strength for Peak Performance,* which presents innovative techniques for developing greater strength and flexibility. His vast knowledge of muscular work dynamics led to his discovery that working the extrinsic ocular muscles can help preserve sight and reeducate the eyes toward better vision. De Angelis came to understand the importance of retinal defocus for transforming ocular refractive status. After thousands of attempts, tests—and mistakes—he proved the power of gradual retinal defocus in preventing and gradually reducing functional refractive errors. Using scientific studies and his personal success in healing his initial refractive error, he hopes to create the basis for a new direction in visual reeducation. De Angelis lives in Rome and can be reached via email at vision@powervisionsystem.com.